Pharmacology in 7 Days for Medical Students

FAZAL-I-AKBAR DANISH

CT2 in Medicine
Princess of Wales Hospital in Bridgend

and

AHMED EHSAN RABBANI

Final Year Medical Student
*Foundation University Medical College (FUMC)
Rawalpindi, Pakistan*

Radcliffe Publishing
Oxford • New York

To my sister and brothers.

Radcliffe Publishing Ltd
18 Marcham Road
Abingdon
Oxon OX14 1AA
United Kingdom

www.radcliffe-oxford.com

Electronic catalogue and worldwide online ordering facility.

British Library Cataloguing in Publication Data

A catalogue record for this book is available from the British Library.

ISBN-13: 978 184619 422 1

The paper used for the text pages of this book
is FSC certified. FSC (The Forest Stewardship
Council) is an international network to promote
responsible management of the world's forests.

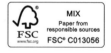

Typeset by Pindar NZ, Auckland, New Zealand
Printed and bound by TJI Digital, Padstow, Cornwall, UK

Contents

Preface

Pharmacology is a volatile subject with a 'very short half-life'. One can cram 20 side effects of a single drug but when one is required to memorise the side effects of 150 drugs, everything gets jumbled up. The same holds true for the lists of therapeutic uses and drug classifications that pharmacology students have to memorise and reproduce in the exam setting. No wonder that many medical students fail in pharmacology not because they haven't 'studied' the subject but simply because they haven't 'retained' the subject matter. This book is written to help solve a very specific and practical problem: how to reproduce the pharmacology subject matter in the exam setting.

First, instead of dividing the syllabus in the conventional way, i.e. 'systems', it is being divided into classifications, mechanisms of action, therapeutic uses, side effects, etc. In the current exam format, it is very unlikely that someone would ask to write an 'essay' on a given drug; instead, very specific questions are asked, like 'give the therapeutic uses of drug "A"', or 'enumerate the side effects of drug "B"', etc. Examiners are more interested in asking, for example, the side effects of chloramphenicol so that students know why this drug is *not* used commonly any more, as compared to the mechanism of action of this drug. Thus, in the chapter on side effects, the side effects of most commonly asked drugs are given; in the chapter on mechanisms of action, the mechanisms of action of most commonly asked drugs are given.

The book may appear deficient in the classical sense – it may contain the side effects of a given drug, with no mention of its mechanism of action or therapeutic uses. But the very aim of writing this book was not to write another treatise of *everything about every drug*, but to 'distil' the information that is directly and specifically relevant to the exams. The book thus truly deserves its title, *Pharmacology in 7 Days for Medical Students*. Students can forget everything they have ever studied about pharmacology in the last seven days prior to the exams, cram this 166-page book and (still) hold a bright chance of passing every and any pharmacology exam.

Fazal-I-Akbar Danish
Ahmed Ehsan Rabbani
January 2010

About the authors

Dr Fazal graduated from Army Medical College, Rawalpindi, Pakistan in 1999. After working in his home country for a few years in various capacities, he came to the UK in 2005. Here he has worked as Clinical Research Fellow in the Universities of Southampton and Bristol, and as a Medical SHO in various NHS trusts. Although a junior doctor, Dr Fazal has contributed appreciably in medical literature. He is the first and corresponding author of eight research papers published in different peer-reviewed journals. He has contributed a 28-web-page section namely 'Phenotyping' in an online encyclopaedia entitled 'Online Encyclopaedia of Genetic Epidemiology Studies', www.oege.org. This section links and describes standardised research protocols and related information for clinical phenotyping on common diseases and risk traits. It is primarily of relevance and consumption of researchers and PhD students. Dr Fazal has three medical books to his credit – the book in your hand, *Hospital Dermatology* (a 226-page book for final-year medical students and postgraduate trainees) and *Essential Lists of Differential Diagnoses for MRCP: with diagnostic hints* (a 272-page book for postgraduate doctors preparing for MRCP (UK) and FCPS (Pakistan) examinations). He is currently working as a CT2 in Medicine at the Princess of Wales Hospital in Bridgend.

Ahmed Ehsan Rabbani is a final-year medical student and the younger brother of Dr Fazal. It was Ahmed who highlighted the need for a pharmacology book that medical students could refer to during the last few days before the exam. To realise his vision, he contributed substantially in the design, literature search, drafting, picture drawing and revision of the manuscript. His most valued contribution is giving his elder brother the all-critical insight regarding what to include and what to exclude in this revision book.

Contributors

Salman S Koul MBBS FCPS-I (Pak) MCPS (Pak)
Registrar
Department of Medicine
Pakistan Institute of Medical Sciences (PIMS)
Islamabad, Pakistan

Fazal R Subhani MBBS FCPS-I (Pak)
Registrar
Department of Pediatrics
Holy Family Hospital
Rawalpindi, Pakistan

Saeeda Yasmin MBBS FCPS (Pak) MRCS (UK)
Consultant Surgeon
Shifa Hospital
Islamabad, Pakistan

1

General pharmacology

Pharmacology

1 Brief definition: Science that deals with drugs.

2 Broad definition: Science that deals with the interaction between living systems and molecules, especially the chemicals introduced from outside the system.

3 Comprehensive definition: Knowledge of history, source, physical and chemical properties; compounding absorption, bio-transformation, distribution, excretion, mechanism of action, structural activity relationship, bio-chemical and physiological effects, and therapeutic/other uses of drugs.

WHO definition of drug

A drug is any substance or product that is used or intended to be used to modify or explore physiological symptoms or pathological states for the benefit of the recipient.

Definition of rational drug therapy

Administration of the right drug indicated for the disease, in the right dose, through an appropriate route of administration, for the right duration.

Criteria for right drug

- Cost-effectiveness
- Efficacy
- Safety

Alkaloids

Characteristics

Mostly solid (rarely liquid), nitrogenous compounds, complex structure, found in plants, intensely bitter in taste, very active biologically, basic in nature and form water-soluble salts with acids, e.g. ephedrine, otherwise insoluble in water (soluble in alcohol). Their names end in the suffix 'ine'.

Examples

Solid alkaloids: Morphine, codeine, ephedrine, atropine, hyoscine, quinine, ergotamine, strychnine.

Liquid alkaloids: Nicotine, lobeline, pilocarpine.

Glycosides
Characteristics
These are an ether-like combination of sugars with organic structure. They are complex-structured, non-nitrogenous compounds found in plants containing C, H and O_2, very active biologically, hydrolysed by acids/enzymes into:

A Sugar portions or glycone.

B Non-sugar portions or aglycone.

When the sugar portion is glucose, it is called glucosides, e.g. salicyclines. Their names end in the suffix 'in'.

Examples
Cardiac glycosides: Like digoxin, digitoxin, gitoxin.

Table 1.1 Differences between fixed and volatile oils

Fixed oils	Volatile oils
Non-volatile	Volatile
Source: animals and plants	Plants alone
They are esters of higher fatty acids	They are hydrocarbons
Insoluble in water	Slightly soluble in water
They give no smell or taste to water	They impart smell and taste to water
They give greasy marks on paper	They do not give greasy marks on paper
They are bland and non-irritant	Mildly irritant
They form soaps with alkalis	They do not form soaps with alkalis
They cannot be distilled without being decomposed	They can be transferred by the process of distillation
They become decomposed and smell rancid when kept for a long time	They do not decompose
They usually have few pharmacological actions, e.g. nutrient and emollient	They have many actions, e.g. carminatives, antiseptics, counter-irritants, expectorants and flavouring agents

Intravenous (I/V) route of administration
Advantages
1 Since absorption is not required, pharmacological action starts instantaneously.

2 Since first-pass metabolism in the liver is bypassed, the bioavailability of intravenously administered drugs is 100%.

3 Valuable for emergency/unconscious patients/patients having vomiting.

4 Permits titration of dosage (increase or decrease the dose).

5 Suitable for large volumes of fluids, blood, plasma and nutrients.

6 Irritant drugs can be given in diluted form.

Disadvantages
1 Drugs once injected cannot be taken out.

2 More risk of side effects like sepsis, phlebitis, etc.

3 Extravasation into the surrounding tissues with resultant possible side effects (like tissue necrosis).

4 Not suitable for oily preparations.

5 Drugs incompatible with blood cannot be given.

6 Because of 100% bioavailability, more vigilant dose titration is required.

Biotransformation
Definition
Biotransformation is a chemical change that a drug undergoes in a living system with consequent change in its solubility and activity.

Objectives
1 Activation of pro-drugs.

2 Inactivation and elimination of drugs.

Advantages of administration of pro-drug
1 To make the drug *more portable*, e.g. chloramphenicol palmitate is given instead of chloramphenicol.

2 To make a drug *tasteless and more stable*, e.g. propoxyphene hydrochloride, which is bitter and unstable, is given in the form of a pro-drug – propoxyphene naphsylate, which is tasteless and stable.

3 To improve the *rate of absorption* of the drug or to remove its toxicity, e.g. talampicillin, pivampicillin and bacampicillin are given instead of ampicillin.

4 To increase the *concentration* of the drug at the site of action, e.g. levodopa instead of dopamine.

5 To increase the *duration of action* of the drug, e.g. in place of phenothiazine, fluphenazine derivatives (like fluphenazine enanthate or fluphenazine decanoate) are given.

Features of mixed function oxidase system (MFOS)
This system is under genetic control. It is inducible and inhabitable. This system has gradually evolved as a result of exposure to toxins in plants and environment. Hence a safety mechanism for humans and animals. Its activity is modified by various factors like age, sex, species, altitude, climate, etc. Cytochrome P450 has multiple isoforms (about 50). Cytochrome P450 enzymes are involved in biotransformation of drugs in human beings.

Drug metabolism and elimination
Drugs are eliminated from human body by two main processes: excretion and metabolism.

   Drug excretion occurs via kidneys, liver or lungs (primarily gaseous anaesthetics). Since renal excretion is the commonest route of drug elimination, in patients with chronic renal impairment, dose reductions become necessary to avoid drug toxicities /side effects. Small amounts of some drugs are excreted in the milk ($\rightarrow$ possible ill effects on the breast-feeding babies).

   Drug metabolism primarily occurs in the liver, especially by the cytochrome P450 (CYP) enzyme system (also called 'microsomal enzymes') embedded in the smooth endoplasmic reticulum. Since polar drugs have poor plasma membrane permeability and thus can't reach the intracellular microsomal enzymes efficiently, most polar drugs are excreted 'unchanged' in the urine. Lipid-soluble drugs on the other hand can cross the plasma membranes and reach the microsomal enzymes very efficiently. Most lipid-soluble drugs thus first undergo metabolism in the liver to more 'polar metabolites' before getting excreted in the urine.

First-pass metabolism: Some drugs are so efficiently metabolised by the hepatic microsomal enzymes that the amount reaching the systemic circulation is much less than the amount absorbed from the gut. This is called first-pass metabolism and the drugs that show extensive first-pass metabolism must be given in larger doses to attain therapeutic levels in the blood when given orally.

Drug metabolites:

1 Parent molecules of some drugs are inactive. They must therefore first undergo metabolism to yield therapeutically active metabolites. For example, azathioprine, an immunosuppressant drug is inactive per se. It first undergoes metabolism to produce mercaptopurine – a therapeutically active metabolite. Such drugs are called *pro-drugs*.

2 Both the parent drug and the metabolite of some drugs are active, though partly dissimilar in their therapeutic effects. For example, aspirin (the parent drug) has both platelet-aggregation inhibition and anti-inflammatory effects. Its metabolite salicylic acid, on the other hand, produces only anti-inflammatory effect.

3 Some drugs, per se, are safe, but their metabolites are toxic and are responsible for the adverse effects of that drug. For example, haemorrhagic cystitis, a very well known side effect of cyclophosphamide is caused by its toxic metabolite (acrolein) and not the parent molecule. Some drugs, per se, are toxic, but their metabolites are safer. For example, terfenadine – a non-sedating antihistamine occasionally causes cardiac arrhythmias, but its active metabolite fexofenadine lacks this side effect. Fexofenadine (the metabolite) has thus replaced terfenadine (the parent drug) in clinical practice.

Enzyme induction and its effects

1 Many drugs induce the hepatic microsomal enzymes. We can imagine that if a patient is getting a drug that is metabolised by microsomal enzymes (e.g. warfarin – an anticoagulant), and he is concomitantly given another drug that induces hepatic microsomal enzymes (e.g. carbamazepine – an anti-epileptic agent), the metabolism of warfarin will increase resulting in a reduction in its therapeutic efficacy. The dose of warfarin must therefore be increased if such a patient needs carbamazepine, or alternatively, an anti-epileptic agent that doesn't induce hepatic microsomal enzymes needs to be prescribed.

2 Besides reducing the therapeutic efficacy of another drug, enzyme induction is sometimes responsible for worsening the side-effect profile of another drug. This is especially true of the drugs that produce toxic metabolites. For example, paracetamol, generally a safe drug is converted to a toxic metabolite called N-acetyl-p-benzoquinone by cytochrome P450 enzyme system. This metabolite is responsible for the hepatic necrosis seen in patients of paracetamol overdose. The risk of potentially life-threatening hepatic necrosis increases if the paracetamol overdose patient has concomitantly taken an enzyme inducer, e.g. alcohol.

3 Many a times the inducing agent itself is a substrate of hepatic microsomal

enzymes, i.e. by inducing these enzymes, the agent increases its own metabolism ($\rightarrow \downarrow$ therapeutic efficacy). Carbamazepine is one such example. It is both an inducer and a substrate of hepatic microsomal enzymes. It is generally given in low doses in the beginning of the therapy to avoid drug toxicity. In the coming few weeks, once the enzymes are induced, higher doses can be tolerated without producing any untoward side effects.

4 In clinical practice, the phenomenon of enzyme induction is sometimes exploited for the benefit of the patient. For example, premature jaundiced babies are prescribed phenobarbitone – an enzyme inducer. This drug, by inducing hepatic glucuronyl-transferase, increases bilirubin conjugation in the hepatocytes with subsequent excretion in the bile. The risk of kernicterus is thus reduced.

Enzyme inhibition and its effects

1 Certain drugs inhibit hepatic microsomal enzymes. If they are coadministered with a drug that is normally metabolised by microsomal enzymes, the metabolism of the latter drug will decrease with consequent increased therapeutic efficacy and/or probability of development of adverse effects. An example is the azathio-prine – allopurinol interaction. As mentioned before, azathioprine (inactive) is metabolised to an active metabolite called mercaptopurine by a hepatic enzyme xanthine oxidase. Allopurinol by inhibiting xanthine oxidase increases the thera-peutic efficacy and potentially the adverse effects probability of azathioprine.

2 In clinical practice, the phenomenon of enzyme inhibition is sometimes exploited for the benefit of the patient. A classical example is that of ethanol-disulfiram interaction. Ethanol (alcohol) is normally metabolised first to acetaldehyde by a hepatic enzyme alcohol dehydrogenase, and then to acetate by aldehyde dehy-drogenase. Disulfiram, a drug used as aversion therapy to discourage people from taking alcohol, inhibits aldehyde dehydrogenase leading to a rise in acetaldehyde concentrations. Acetaldehyde produces extremely unpleasant (though not harmful) effects including tachycardia, hyperventilation, flushing and panic. Metronidazole, an antimicrobial agent also inhibits aldehyde dehydrogenase enzyme and thus patients on metronidazole therapy are advised to avoid alcohol for the duration of the therapy.

Tolerance

Tolerance is defined as 'unusual resistance to a drug causing either a total loss or a decreased response to a drug'.

Types

1 *Pseudo-tolerance*: is defined as 'resistance to drug response on oral route of admin-istration only, if a drug is taken for a long time in small amounts'.

2 *True-tolerance*: is defined as 'resistance to drug response on both oral/parenteral route of administration'. It could be:
    a Natural (species or racial).
    b Acquired (functional or dispositional).

3 *Cross-tolerance*: means 'if tolerance develops in an individual to one member of a group of drugs, then tolerance will also be seen with other members of that group'. *Example*: Opioids: If an individual show tolerance to morphine, then he will also show tolerance to pethidine.

4 *Tissue-tolerance*: Means 'certain drugs produce tolerance limited to certain tissues/ organs, while other tissues/organs are spared'.

Example: Morphine: Tolerance develops to its analgesic, euphoric, sedative and hypnotic effects; but not with the myotic, pleuritic and constipating effects.

Tachyphylaxis
Definition
It means acute tolerance that develops rapidly, when certain indirectly acting sympathomimetic drugs like amphetamine, ephedrine and tyramine, etc. are administered to humans/animals repeatedly in short intervals.

Table 1.2 **Differences between tolerance and tachyphylaxis**

Tolerance	Tachyphylaxis
It develops slowly, when certain drugs are administered over prolonged periods	It develops rapidly, when certain drugs are given at short intervals of time
It develops with directly-acting drugs like barbiturates, benzodiazepines, opioids and alcohol	It develops with indirectly acting sympathomimetics like amphetamine, ephedrine and tyramine
Directly acting drugs act directly on the target organ on the specific receptors	It develops when indirectly acting drugs deplete the stores of biogenic amines in adrenergic nerve terminals
Remedy: By increasing the dose of directly acting drugs, biological effects can be achieved	Remedy: Increasing the dose cannot produce biological response. It's only the drug holiday that causes repletion of noradrenergic stores to produce biological effects

Idiosyncrasy
Definition
It is qualitatively abnormal response to certain drugs.

Characteristics
1 It is highly unpredictable – can occur even after the first dose of the drug.
2 It has got a genetic basis – abnormality in the genes that control receptors/drug-metabolising enzymes/cellular metabolism.
3 It could be fatal.

Examples
Some of the drugs causing idiosyncratic reactions include:
1 Chloramphenicol: as an idiosyncratic reaction, chloramphenicol can cause aplastic anaemia.
2 Sodium valproate: can cause hepatotoxicity.
3 Halothane and suxamethonium: can cause malignant hyperthermia.

Synergism
Definition
Synergism is a form of pharmacological cooperation between two drugs in which two drugs with similar pharmacological effects on the biological system when

coadministered lead to an increase in the final effect of each drug.

Types: Two types: summation and potentiation.

1 *Summation*: is a type of synergism in which the final effect of the two drugs given together is equal to the algebraic sum of individual effects of these drugs.

Examples:
- General anaesthetics: Chloroform and ether – both general anaesthetics when coadministered lead to augmented effect by a process of summation.
- Use of ephedrine and aminophylline in bronchial asthma.

2 *Potentiation*: is a form of synergism where final effect on the biological system is more than the algebraic sum of individual effects of the two drugs.

Example: Cotrimoxazole contains two drugs, sulphamethaxazole and trimethoprim. These two drugs potentiate each other's pharmacological effects. When coadministered, the antibacterial spectrum of the individual drugs broadens. Thus more efficacy can be achieved with lesser dosage. The incidence of toxicity is also reduced in this way.

Antagonism
Definition
It is the opposing effects of two drugs on the biological system when given together. It is a sort of pharmacological non-cooperation between the two drugs. By antagonism the final effect is decreased/totally abolished/reversed.

Types: Three types: chemical, physiological and pharmacological.

1 *Chemical antagonism*: In chemical antagonism, one drug abolishes the effect of other drug by chemical reaction.

Example: Antacids: like sodium bicarbonate, aluminium hydroxide and magnesium hydroxide are given in hyperacidity states like peptic ulcer.

Whereas aluminium hydroxide when given alone causes constipation, and magnesium hydroxide when given alone causes diarrhoea, coadministration of aluminium hydroxide and magnesium hydroxide leads to neither constipation nor diarrhoea. Chemical reaction between $NaHCO_3$ and HCl:

$$NaHCO_3 + HCl \rightarrow NaCl + H_2O + CO_2$$

So HCl is destroyed in stomach by $NaHCO_3$ by a process of chemical antagonism.

2 *Physiological antagonism*: In physiological antagonism, two drugs given together oppose/reverse/abolish the effect of one drug by acting independently on the specific receptors by their own separate mechanism of action.

Example: Adrenaline vs histamine in anaphylactic shock: In anaphylactic shock, histamine is released from pre-sensitised mast cells when certain drug is given for the second time. Histamine acts on its own H1 receptors on the blood vessels and bronchial muscle causing vasodilatation, increased vascular permeability and bronchoconstriction. The net effect is fall in blood pressure and respiratory distress. Adrenaline has opposite effects on blood vessels and bronchial muscle – it causes vasoconstriction (by acting on α receptors) and bronchodilatation (by acting on $\beta2$ receptors).

3 *Pharmacological antagonism*: In pharmacological antagonism, two drugs acting on the same receptors in a biological system – one as agonist and other as antagonist – when coadministered compete with each other for receptor attachment.

Types: Two types: competitive (reversible) and non-competitive (irreversible).

Competitive (reversible) antagonism: In this, by increasing the concentration of agonist at the receptor site, we can reverse/displace the antagonist from the receptor site. *Example*: Atropine vs acetylcholine at muscarinic receptors; morphine vs nalaxone at opioid receptors.

Non-competitive (irreversible) antagonism: In this, by increasing the concentration of agonist at the receptor site, we cannot reverse/displace the antagonist because the antagonist forms a very firm covalent bond with the receptor, which cannot be broken down by increasing the concentration of agonist at the receptor site.

Example: Phenoxybenzamine vs noradrenalin at α receptors.

Allergy

An allergy is a qualitatively abnormal response to some drugs/vaccines/antisera/dust/pollens/various food stuff/various animal food products in sensitised (atopic) individuals having immunological basis. It is mediated by IgE directed against a specific antigen and located over the cell surface of mast cells. On antigen exposure, the antigen-IgE adhesion leads to mast cell degranulation with resultant liberation of inflammatory mediators like histamine, which mediate an acute inflammatory response including vasodilatation and bronchospasm.

These allergic hypersensitivity reactions could be mild, not requiring drug therapy. Examples include drug fever, skin eruptions like urticaria, allergic rhinitis/hayfever, allergic conjunctivitis, food allergy resulting in diarrhoea.

The manifestations of allergy depend upon the tissue exposed to the allergen. Mild manifestations are short-lived.

Severe/fatal allergic reactions include anaphylactic shock.

Delayed allergic reactions (called serum sickness): It manifests in the form of eruptions, lymphadenopathy, joint pains and fever. It is mediated through T-lymphocytes (also known as cell-mediated immunity).

Anaphylaxis
Definition

A rapidly developing immunological reaction occurring within minutes after the combination of an antigen with an antibody bound to mast cells or basophils in individuals or animals previously sensitised to the antigen.

Chemical mediators of anaphylaxis

Histamine, 5HT, slow-reacting substance of anaphylaxis (SRS-A), eosinophilic chemotactic factor of anaphylaxis (ECF-A), prostaglandins, platelet-activating factor, and kinins.

Treatment of anaphylaxis

- *First-line drug: adrenaline* 1:1000 solution 0.3–0.5 mL I/M, if patient is in shock (never I/V because it causes potentially fatal ventricular fibrillation).
- *Second-line drugs*:
    - *Corticosteroids* (hydrocortisone sodium succinate 100 mg I/V or dexamethasone up to 4 mg I/V, followed by prednisolone 50–100 mg orally in divided doses).
    - *Antihistamines*: promethazine HCl 0.5–1 mg/kg I/V or diphenhydramine 50–100 mg I/V.

- *Miscellaneous drugs:* aminophylline 6 mg/kg I/V or metaraminol 1.5–5 mg I/V.
- *Supportive treatment:* I/V fluids, oxygen, tracheostomy, endotracheal intubation.

Drugs that can cause anaphylaxis

Horse serum, penicillins, cephalosporins, plasma expanders (dextran; polygeline), parenteral vitamin B complex, aminoglycosides, amphotericin B, L-asparaginase.

WHO definition of drug dependence

Drug dependence is a psychological or sometimes physical state resulting from the interaction between a living organism and a drug, characterised by behavioural and other responses that always include a compulsion to take the drug on a continuous or periodic basis in order to experience its psychological/ physical effects and sometimes to avoid the discomfort of its absence.

Tolerance may or may not be present. A person may be dependent on more than one drug.

Components of drug dependence

Euphoria, tolerance, psychological/physical dependence and withdrawal syndrome.

Drugs causing drug dependence

Drugs causing severe psychological or physical dependence: Examples include morphine, codeine, pethidine, methadone, benzodiazepine, barbiturates, amphetamines and ethyl alcohol.
Drugs causing psychological dependence only: Examples include cocaine, cannabis, nicotine, caffeine and LSD.

Management of drug dependence

1 Gradual or sudden withdrawal of the drug.
2 Substitution therapy.
3 Specific drug therapy.
4 Psychotherapy.
5 Occupational therapy.
6 Correction of nutritional deficiencies.
7 Community treatment and rehabilitation.

Bioavailability of drugs

'Bioavailability' means availability of a biologically active drug in a biologic system, especially at the site of action. It is the fraction of the drug/dose of the drug that reaches the systemic circulation in unchanged active form after administration by any route of a pharmaceutical preparation containing that active drug.

Factors affecting bioavailability

1 Quality control in manufacturing and formulation.
2 All factors affecting absorption of the drug from the GIT.
3 First pass metabolism.

Dose-response curve

It is the graphical representation of the relationship between the dose of a drug and the response to a drug within a biological system.

Types

Graded dose-response curve: It is the quantitative curve in which increasing doses of a drug produces varying changes and effects.

Quantal dose-response curve: It is a curve that describes the distribution of minimum doses that produce a given effect in a population of test animals.

Cumulative dose-response curve: The numbers of determination are cumulatively added until all are accounted for.

Median effective dose: It is the dose of a drug required to produce a specified intensity of effect in 50% of the individuals. It is abbreviated as ED_{50}.

Median lethal dose: It is the dose of a drug required to kill 50% of experimented animals. It is abbreviated as LD_{50}. It is the measure to toxicity of a drug.

Therapeutic index (TI): It is the ratio of LD_{50} to $ED_{50.}$

$$TI = LD_{50}/ED_{50.}$$

Plasma half-life (t½)

Definition

It is the time required for the concentration of a drug in the plasma to decrease to one-half of its initial value after the steady state plasma concentration has been achieved.

$$t\frac{1}{2} = \frac{0.7 \times Vd}{CL}$$

Vd: volume of distribution; CL: clearance of drug.

$$CL = \frac{\text{rate of elimination of drug}}{\text{plasma drug concentration}}$$

Factors affecting t½

1 Type of kinetics – zero or first order.
2 Enzyme inhibitors ($\rightarrow \downarrow$ metabolism $\rightarrow \uparrow$ plasma t½).
3 Enzyme inducers ($\rightarrow \uparrow$ metabolism $\rightarrow \downarrow$ t½).
4 Active metabolites ($\rightarrow \uparrow$ t½ of a drug).
5 Enterohepatic recirculation of a drug ($\rightarrow \uparrow$ t½).
6 Diseases of organs of elimination – liver and kidney ($\uparrow$ t½).
7 Changes in the rate of blood flow to organs of elimination – liver and kidney.
8 Displacement of drug from plasma protein binding (PPB) sites ($\uparrow$ Vd $\rightarrow \uparrow$ t½).

2

Classifications

Adrenergic drugs
A Chemical classification
  1 Catecholamines
    i Natural
- Adrenaline
- Dopamine
- Noradrenaline

    ii Synthetic
- Dobutamine
- Isoetherine
- Isoprenaline
- Hexaprenaline
- Rimiterol

  2 Non-catecholamines
- Amphetamine
- Dexamphetamine
- Ephedrine
- Metaraminol
- Pseudoephedrine
- Terbutaline

B Classification based on mechanism of action
  1 Both directly and indirectly acting sympathomimetics
- Ephedrine
- Metaraminol

  2 Directly acting sympathomimetics
- Adrenaline
- Isoprenaline
- Noradrenaline
- Salbutamol
- Terbutaline

  3 Indirectly acting sympathomimetics
    i Release of noradrenaline
- Amphetamine
- Methylamphetamine
- Tyramine

    ii Reuptake inhibitors

- Cocaine
- Tricyclic antidepressants

C **Classification based on receptor selectivity**
  1 **Mainly α-receptor agonists**
    i **α1-agonists**
- Methoxamine
- Phenylephrine
- Xylometazoline

    ii **α2-agonists**
- α-methyldopa
- Clonidine

    iii **α1 and α2 combined agonists**
- Oxymetazoline

  2 **Mainly β-receptor agonists**
    i **β1 agonists**
- Dobutamine
- Prenalterol

    ii **β2 agonists**
- Fenterol
- Ritodrine
- Salbutamol
- Terbutaline

    iii **Selective β1 and β2 agonists**
- Isoprenaline
- Orciprenaline

  3 **α and β agonists**
- Adrenaline
- Amphetamine
- Ephedrine
- Noradrenaline

  4 **Adrenergic and dopaminergic agonists**
- Dopamine

Cephalosporin generations (classification based on spectrum of antimicrobial activity)

1st Generation
- Cephalexin
- Cephradine
- Cefadroxil
- Cefazolin

2nd Generation
- Cefaclor
- Cefamandole
- Cefprozil
- Cefoxitin
- Cefuroxime

3rd Generation
- Cefixime

- Cefoperazone
- Ceftazidime
- Ceftizoxime
- Ceftriaxone

4th Generation
- Cefepime

Chemical classification of antidepressants (TCA)

1 Dibenzepines
- Imipramine
- Desipramine
- Trimipramine

2 Dibenzoxepine
- Doxepine

3 Dibenzoxazepine
- Amoxapine

4 Dibenzocycloheptadienes
- Amitriptyline
- Nortriptyline

5 Dibenzocycloheptatriene
- Protriptyline

6 Miscellaneous
- Maprotiline

Chemical classification of anti-epileptic drugs

1 Long-acting barbiturates
- Phenobarbitone
- Methyl phenobarbitone

2 Deoxybarbiturates
- Primidone

3 Benzodiazepines
- Diazepam
- Clonazepam
- Lorazepam
- Nitrazepam

4 Hydantoin derivatives
- Phenytoin
- Mephenytoin
- Ethotoin

5 Valproic acid derivatives
- Valproic acid
- Sodium valproate

6 Iminostilbines
- Carbamazepine
- Oxcarbamazepine

7 Succinimides
- Ethosuximide
- Phensuximide

Newer drugs:
1 GABA analogue
- Gabapentin
- Vigabatrin

2 Miscellaneous
- Lamotrigine
- Felbamate
- Topiramate

Older drugs:
1 Bromides
- Sodium and Potassium bromide

2 Carbonic anhydrase inhibitors
- Acetazolamide

3 Oxazolidinedione derivatives
- Trimethadione

4 Miscellaneous
- Paraldehyde

Adrenocorticosteroids

Natural
1 Glucocorticoids
- Cortisol
- Corticosterone

2 Mineralocorticoids
- Aldosterone
- 11-Deoxy corticosterone acetate

Synthetic
1 Glucocorticoids
- Cortisone
- Prednisone
- Prednisolone
- Methylprednisolone
- Paramethasone
- Dexamethasone
- Triamcinolone
- Betamethasone valerate
- Beclomethasone dipropionate

2 Mineralocorticoids
1 Fludrocortisone

Antiviral drugs

1 Agents to treat herpes simplex virus (HSV) and varicella-zoster virus (VSV) infections (DNA-polymerase inhibitors)
- Acyclovir
- Valacyclovir
- Famciclovir

- Penciclovir
- Foscarnet
- Trifluridine

2 Agents to treat cytomegalovirus (CMV) infections
- Cidofovir
- Foscarnet
- Fomivirsen
- Ganciclovir
- Valganciclovir

3 Antiretroviral agents
  i Nucleoside reverse transcriptase inhibitors (NRTIs)
  - Abacavir
  - Didanosine
  - Lamivudine
  - Stavudine
  - Zidovudine
  - Zalcitabine

  ii Non-nucleoside reverse transcriptase inhibitors (NNRTIs)
  - Delavirdine
  - Efavirenz
  - Nevirapine

  iii Protease inhibitors
  - Amprenavir
  - Indinavir
  - Nelfinavir
  - Ritonavir
  - Saquinavir

  iv Fusion inhibitors
  - Enfuvirtide

4 Antihepatitis agents
- Adefovir
- Interferon
- Lamivudine
- Ribavirin

5 Anti-influenza agents
- Amantadine
- Rimantadine
- Oseltamivir
- Zanamivir

NSAIDs
A Drugs with analgesic and marked anti-inflammatory effects
  1 Salicylic acid derivatives
  - Aspirin (acetyl salicylic acid)
  - Salicylic acid
  - Sodium salicylate
  - Methyl salicylate
  - Choline salicylate

- Magnesium salicylate
- Diflunisal
- Benorylate

2 **Pyrazolone derivatives**
- Phenylbutazone
- Oxyphenbutazone
- Azapropazone

3 **Acetic acid derivatives**
- Diclofenac
- Indomethacin
- Tolmetin
- Sulnidac
- Etodolac

4 **Oxicams**
- Piroxicam
- Meloxicam

5 **Miscellaneous**
- Nimuselide
- Celecoxib
- Rofecoxib

B **Drugs with analgesic and moderate anti-inflammatory effects**
1 **Propionic acid derivatives**
- Ibuprofen
- Ketoprofen
- Fenoprofen
- Flurbiprofen
- Carprofen
- Indoprofen
- Naproxen
- Oxaprozin

2 **Fenamic acid derivatives**
- Mefenamic acid
- Meclofenamic acid
- Flufenamic acid
- Tolfenamic acid

C **Drugs with analgesic and weak anti-inflammatory effects**
- Paracetamol (aniline derivative)

Adrenergic neuron blockers

1 **Drugs which interfere with synthesis of noradrenaline**
- Metyrosine (alpha-methyl tyrosine)

2 **Drugs that inhibit storage of noradrenaline**
- Deserpidine
- Reserpine

3 **Drugs that prevent release of noradrenaline**
- Bethanidine
- Debrisoquin
- Guanadrel

- Guanethidine
- Guanoxan

Alpha-adrenergic blockers
A **Chemical classification**
  1 **Beta-haloalkylamines**
     - Dibenamine
     - Phenoxybenzamine
  2 **Benzodioxans**
     - Dibuzaine
     - Diperoxan
  3 **Benzene sulfonamide**
     - Tamsulosin
  4 **Dibenzapines**
     - Azepetine
  5 **Ergot alkaloid**
     - Dihydroergotamine
     - Ergotamine
  6 **Phenothiazines**
     - Chlorpromazine
  7 **Phenoxyalkylamines**
     - Thymoxamine
  8 **Piperazinyl quinazolines**
     - Doxazosin
     - Prazosin
     - Terazosin
  9 **Substituted imidazolines**
     - Phentolamine
     - Tolazoline
  10 **Miscellaneous**
     - Carvedilol
     - Indoramin
     - Labetalol
B **According to reversibility of action**
  1 **Irreversible (non-competitive blockers; long-acting)**
     - Dibenamine
     - Phenoxybenzamine
  2 **Reversible (competitive blockers; short-acting)**
     - Doxazosin
     - Prazosin
     - Phentolamine
     - Terazosin
     - Tolazoline
     - Trimazosin
     - Urapidil
C **According to receptor selectivity**
  1 **Mixed α and β adrenoceptor blocking drugs**
     - Carvedilol

- Labetalol
2 **Selective α-blockers**
  i **α1-blockers**
    - Alfuzosin
    - Doxazosin
    - Pinacidal
    - Prazosin
    - Tamsulosin
    - Teruzosin
    - Trimazosin
  ii **α2-blockers**
    - Idazoxan
    - Yohimbine
3 **Non-selective (both α1 and α2-blockers)**
  - Dibenamine
  - Dihydroergotamine
  - Ergotamine
  - Phentolamine
  - Phenoxybenzamine
  - Tolazoline

Aminoglycosides
1 **Natural**
  - Gentamycin
  - Kanamycin
  - Neomycin
  - Streptomycin
  - Tobramycin
2 **Semi-synthetic**
  - Amikacin
  - Netilmicin

Members of macrolide group
- Azithromycin
- Clarithromycin
- Roxithromycin
- Telithromycin
- Carbomycin
- Erythromycin
- Oleandomycin
- Spiramycin

Amoebicides
A **Chemical classification**
  1 **Dichloroacetamides**
    - Clefamide
    - Etofamide
    - Diloxanide furoate

- Teclozan
2 **Emetines**
   - Emetine
   - Dehydroemetine
3 **Nitroimidazoles**
   - Metronidazole
   - Ornidazole
   - Tinidazole
4 **Halogenated hydroxyquinolines**
   - Broxyquinoline
   - Clioquinol (Iodochlorohydroxyquin)
   - Iodoquinol (Diiodohydroxyquin)
5 **Chloroquine**
6 **Antibiotics**
   - Erythromycin
   - Paromomycin
   - Tetracyclines
B **Therapeutic classification**
   1 **Tissue amoebicides**
      a **Emetines**
         - Emetine
         - Dehydroemetine
      b **Nitroimidazoles**
         - Metronidazole
         - Ornidazole
         - Tinidazole
      c **Chloroquine**
   2 **Luminal amoebicides**
      a **Dichloroacetamides**
         - Clefamide
         - Etofamide
         - Diloxanide furoate
         - Teclozan
      b **Halogenated hydroxyquinolines**
         - Broxyquinoline
         - Clioquinol (iodochlorohydroxyquin)
         - Iodoquinol (diiodohydroxyquin)
      c **Antibiotics**
         - Erythromycin
         - Paromomycin
         - Tetracyclines

Anti-anginal drugs
1 **β-adrenoceptor blockers**
   - Atenolol
   - Acebutalol
   - Propranolol
2 **Calcium channel blockers**

    a **Benzothiazepine**
- Diltiazem

    b **Diarylaminopropylamine**
- Bepridil

    c **Dihydropyridines**
- Amlodipine
- Fenodipine
- Nicardipine
- Nifedipine
- Nimodipine
- Nisoldipine
- Nitrendipine

    d **Diphenylpiperazines**
- Flunarizine
- Ranolazine
- Trimetazidine

    e **Phenyl Alkylamines**
- Gallopamil
- Verapamil

3 Organic nitrates and nitrites

    a **Intermediate-acting**
- Isosorbide dinitrate (chewable oral)
- Nitroglycerin (2% ointment; slow-release buccal)

    b **Long-acting**
- Erythrityl tetranitrate
- Isosorbide-5-mononitrate (oral)
- Nitroglycerin (oral sustained action; slow release patch)

    c **Short-acting**
- Amylnitrite (inhalant)
- Isosorbide dinitrate (sublingual)
- Nitroglycerin (sublingual)

4 Potassium channel activators
- Cromakalin
- Nicorandil
- Pinacidil

Anti-asthmatic drugs

I Bronchodilators

    A **Antimuscarinics**
- Ipratropium bromide
- Tiotropium

    B **Methylxanthines**
- Aminophylline
- Caffeine
- Theobromine
- Theophylline

    C **Sympathomimetics**

       i α and β-adrenoceptor agonists

- Epinephrine
- Ephedrine
- Isoproterenol

ii **β-adrenoceptor agonists**
- Isoprenaline
- Orciprenaline

iii **β2-Selective adrenoceptor agonists**
- Formoterol
- Remiterol
- Salbutamol
- Terbutaline

II Corticosteroids
- Beclomethasone
- Dexamethasone
- Hydrocortisone Sodium Succinate
- Methyl Prednisolone
- Triamcinolone

III Leukotriene pathway inhibitors
a **LTD4-receptor antagonists**
- Montelukast
- Zafirlukast

b **5-lipoxygenase inhibitor**
- Zileuton

IV Mast cell stabilisers/degranulation inhibitors
- Disodium cromoglycate/cromolyn sodium
- Ketotifen
- Nedocromil sodium

V New approaches
a **Anti-IgE monoclonal antibodies**
- Omalizumab

b **Ca2+ channel blockers**
- Nifedipine
- Verapamil

Parasympatholytics/cholinolytics/anticholinergic drugs
A Chemical classification
1 **Natural**
- Atropine
- Hyoscine (scopolamine)

2 **Synthetic and semi-synthetic**
i **Tertiary amines**
- Dicyclomine
- Homatropine
- Pirenzepine
- Tropicamide

ii **Quartenary amines**
- Atropine methobromide
- Glycopyrrolate

- Ipratropium bromide
- Propantheline bromide
- Pipenzolate bromide

B Therapeutic classification

  1 Anti-asthmatics
- Ipratropium bromide
- Tiotropium

  2 Antidote to cholinergic poisoning
- Atropine sulphate

  3 Antidiarrhoeal
- Atropine sulphate
- Diphenoxylate

  4 Anti-Parkinsonism
- Benzhexol
- Benztropine
- Biperidine
- Orphenadine
- Procyclidine

  5 Antispasmodic
- Atropine sulphate
- Clidineum bromide
- Hyoscine butylbromide
- Pipenzolate bromide

  6 Anti-ulcer
- Pirenzepine
- Telenzepine

  7 As pre-anaesthetic medication and in motion sickness
- Atropine sulphate
- Hyoscine butylbromide

  8 Mydriatics and cycloplegics
- Atropine sulphate
- Cyclopentolate hydrochloride
- Eucatropine hydrochloride
- Homatropine hydrobromide
- Tropicamide

Anticoagulants

1 Used in vivo and in vitro
- Heparin

2 Used in vivo only

  a Coumarin derivatives
- Dicumarol
- Nicoumalone
- Warfarin

  b Indandione derivatives
- Anisindione
- Diphenindione
- Phenindione

3 Used in vitro only: oxalates and citrates of Na^+ and K^+, e.g.
- EDTA (ethylene diamine tetra-acetic acid)
- Hirudine
- K-Oxalate
- Na-Oxalate

4 Miscellaneous
- Human antithrombin-III
- Lepirudin

Thrombolytic drugs

These include
1 Alteplase
2 Anistreplase
3 Reteplase
4 Streptokinase
5 Tenecteplase
6 Tissue plasminogen activator
7 Urokinase

Antidepressant drugs

1 Tricyclic antidepressants (TCA)
- Imipramine
- Desipramine
- Trimipramine
- Amitriptyline
- Protriptyline
- Nortriptyline

2 Monoamine oxidase inhibitors (MAOI)

  a Hydrazides
- Phenelzine
- Isocarboxazid
- Iproniazid

  b Non-hydrazides
- Tranylcypromine
- Paragyline

3 Selective serotonin reuptake inhibitors (SSRI)
- Sertraline
- Fluoxetine
- Paroxetine

4 Heterocyclic/2nd and 3rd generation antidepressants

  a Monocyclic drugs
- Tofanacine

  b Bicyclic drugs
- Viloxazine

  c Tricyclic drugs
- Amoxapine

  d Tetracyclic drugs
- Maprotiline

23

  e **Others**
  - Bupropion
  - Trazodone
5 **Miscellaneous**
  - Alprazolam
  - Flupenthixol

Antidiarrhoeal drugs

1 **Antimotility agents (drugs that prolong intestinal transit time by reducing motility)**
  a **Anticholinergics**
    - Atropine
    - Dicyclomine HCl
    - Propantheline
  b **Bismuth subsalicylate**
  c **Naturally occurring opium alkaloids**
    - Codeine phosphate
  d **Synthetic opioid compounds**
    - Diphenoxylate
    - Loperamide
2 **Adsorbants**
  - Chalk
  - Charcoal
  - Isphagol husk
  - Kaolin
  - Methyl cellulose
  - Pectin
3 **Miscellaneous**
  - Peppermint oil
  - Vegetable astringent

Anti-emetics

1 **Anticholinergics**
  - Hyoscine
2 **Antihistamines (H_1-antagonists)**
  - Cyclizine
  - Hydroxyzine
  - Meclizine
  - Promethazine
  - Dimenhydrinate
  - Diphenhydramine
3 **Benzodiazepines**
  - Diazepam
4 **Cannabinoids**
  - Dronabinol
  - Nabilone
5 **D2-receptor antagonists**
  - Domperidone

- Metoclopramide
6 Glucocorticoids
- Dexamethasone
- Methylprednisolone
7 Neurokinin-I-receptor-antagonists
- Aprepitant
8 Phenothiazines
- Chlorpromazine
- Prochlorperazine
- Thiethylperazine
9 Selective 5-HT3 receptor antagonists
- Dolasetron
- Granisetron
- Ondansetron
- Palonosetron

Antifungal drugs
1 Drugs that disrupt fungal cell membrane
  A Polyenes
- Amphotericin
- Nystatin
  B Azoles
    i Imidazoles
- Ketoconazole
    ii Triazoles
- Fluconazole
    iii Allylamines
- Terbinafine
2 Drug that inhibits mitosis
- Griseofulvin
3 Drug that inhibits DNA synthesis
- Flucytosine

Antimalarial drugs
A Chemical classification
  1 Cinchona alkaloids
- Quinine
  2 Diaminopyrimidine
- Pyrimethamine
  3 Folate antagonists
- Proguanil
  4 4-Aminoquinolines
- Amodiaquine
- Chloroquine
  5 8-Aminoquinolines
- Primaquine
  6 Quinoline methanol
- Mefloquine

- Quinidine
7 Sulfonamides
  - Sulphadoxine
8 Sulphones
  - Dapsone
9 Tetracyclines
  - Doxycycline
10 Miscellaneous
  - Halofantrin
  - Qinghaosu derivatives (artemisinins), i.e. artemether and artisunate
11 Combinations
  - Fansidar (pyrimethamine + sulfadoxine)
  - Fansimef (pyrimethamine + sulfadoxine + mefloquine)
  - Maloprim (pyrimethamine + dapsone)
  - Malarone (atovaquone + proguanil)
B Classification based on site of action
  1 Tissue schizonticides (acting on hepatic cycle: pre-erythrocytic stage)
    a Against primary tissue forms for causal prophylaxis
      - Proguanil
    b Against latent tissue forms, for terminal prophylaxis/radical cure
      - Primaquine
  2 Blood schizonticides (acting on erythrocytic cycle for suppressive cure)
    a Rapidly acting blood schizonticides
      - Artemisinins
      - Amodiaquine
      - Chloroquine
      - Halofantrin
      - Mefloquine
      - Quinine
    b Slower acting blood schizonticides
      - Doxycycline
      - Proguanil
      - Pyrimethamine
  3 Gametocides against sexual erythrocytic forms
    - Primaquine (against plasmodium falciparum)
    - Chloroquine and quinine (against plasmodium vivax and ovale)

Antigout drugs
A Drugs for acute attack
  1 Natural alkaloids
    - Colchicine
    - Demecolchicine
  2 NSAIDs specially used in gout
    - Fenoprofen
    - Indomethacine
    - Naproxen
    - Oxaprozin
    - Oxyphenbutazone

- Phenylbutazone
- Piroxicam

3 **Corticosteroids**
  - Hydrocortisone
  - Prednisolone

B **Drugs for chronic gout**
  1 **Drugs which increase excretion of uric acid (uricosuric agents)**
     - Aspirin (in high doses)
     - Oxyphenbutazone
     - Phenylbutazone
     - Probenecid
     - Sulfinpyrazone
  2 **Drugs which decrease synthesis of uric acid (xanthine oxidase inhibitors)**
     - Allopurinol

Antihelminthic drugs

1 **Drugs acting against nematodes**
   - Albendazole
   - Mebendazole
   - Thiabendazole
   - Diethyl carbamazine
   - Pyrantel pamoate

2 **Drugs acting against trematodes**
   - Praziquantel

3 **Drugs acting against cestodes**
   - Niclosamide

Drugs used in the Rx of leprosy

- Clofazimine
- Dapsone
- Fluoroquinolones
- Macrolides
- Minocycline
- Rifampicin
- Miscellaneous:
  - Ethionamide
  - Thalidomide

Drugs used in the Rx of tuberculosis

1 **First-line drugs**
   - Ethambutol
   - Isoniazid
   - Pyrazinamide
   - Rifampin
   - Streptomycin

2 **Second-line drugs**
   - Alikacin and kanamycin

- Ciprofloxacin, levofloxacin and ofloxacin
- Capreomycin
- Cycloserine
- Ethionamide
- Rifabutin
- Rifapentine

Antihypertensive drugs

A Calcium channel blockers

  1 Benzothiazepines
- Diltiazem

  2 Diarylaminopropylamine
- Bepridil

  3 Dihydropyridines
- Amlodipine
- Felodipine
- Isradipine
- Nicardipine
- Nifedipine
- Nimodipine
- Nisoldipine
- Nitrendipine

  4 Diphenylpiperazines
- Flunarizine
- Ranolazine
- Trimetazidine

  5 Phenyl Alkylamines
- Gallopamil
- Verapamil

B Diuretics

  1 Loop diuretics
- Bumetanide
- Ethacrynic acid
- Furosemide

  2 Potassium-sparing diuretics
- Amiloride
- Spironolactone
- Triamterene

  3 Thiazides and related agents
- Benzthiazide
- Chlorthalidone
- Chlorothiazide
- Hydrochlorothiazide
- Indapamide

C Drugs acting on renin-angiotensin system

  1 Angiotensin converting enzyme (ACE) inhibitors
- Benzapril
- Captopril

- Enalapril
- Lisinopril
- Perindopril
- Quinapril

2 **Angiotensin II receptor blockers (competitive antagonists)**
- Candesartan
- Eprosartan
- Irbesartan
- Losartan
- Sarasalin
- Telmisartan
- Valsartan

D Sympathoplegics

1 **α and β blockers**
- Carvedilol
- Labetalol

2 **α-adrenergic receptor antagonists**
- Doxazosin
- Phentolamine
- Phenoxybenzmine
- Prazosin
- Terazosin

3 **Adrenergic neuron blockers**
- Guanethidine
- Reserpine

4 **β-adrenergic receptor antagonists**
- Atenolol
- Metoprolol
- Propranolol

5 **Centrally acting drugs**
- Clonidine
- Guanabenz
- Guanfacine
- Methyldopa

6 **Ganglion-blocking drugs**
- Trimethaphan

E Vasodilators

1 **Arterial and venous**
- Sodium nitroprusside

2 **Arterial**
  i **Oral**
  - Hydralazine
  - Minoxidil
  ii **Parenteral**
  - Diazoxide
  - Fenoldopam

3 **Venodilators**
- Nitroglycerin

Anti-Parkinsonian drugs
1 Dopaminergic drugs
- a Dopamine precursors
  - Levodopa
- b Dopadecarboxylase inhibitors
  - Carbidopa
  - Benserazide
- c Dopamine releasing drugs
  - Amantadine

2 Dopaminergic agonist drugs
- a Ergot derivatives
  - Bromocriptine
  - Pergolide
- b Non-ergot derivatives
  - Pramipexole
  - Ropinirole

3 MAO-B inhibitors
- Selegiline
- Rasagiline

4 Selective COMT (catechol-O-methyl transferase) inhibitors
- Tolcapone
- Entacapone

5 Centrally acting antimuscarinics
- Biperidine
- Benzotropine
- Benzhexol
- Procyclidine
- Orphenadrine

6 Other new approaches
- a Gene therapy
- b Surgery
  - Implantation of dopamine rich fragments of tissues, e.g. brain, adrenal glands.
  - Thalomotomy
  - Pallidotomy
  - Thalamic stimulation by implanted electrodes
- c Free radical scavengers
  - Vitamin 'E'

Antipeptic ulcer drugs
1 Antacids
- a Systemic
  - Sodium bicarbonate
- b Non-systemic
  - i Chemically acting
    - Bismuth subcarbonate
    - Calcium carbonate
    - Magnesium carbonate

- Magnesium hydroxide
- Magnesium oxide

   ii **Physically acting**
  - Anion exchange resins
  - Milk and mucin

   iii **Physico-chemically acting**
  - Aluminium hydroxide
  - Aluminium phosphate
  - Magnesium trisilicate

2 Anticholinergics

  a **Natural alkaloids**
  - Atropine
  - Hyoscine

  b **Semi-synthetic**
  - Hyoscine butylbromide

  c **Selective anticholinergic**
  - Pirenzepine

  d **Synthetic**

   i **Quartenary ammonium compounds**
  - Pipenzolate
  - Propantheline

   ii **Tertiary amines**
  - Dicyclomine
  - Piperidolate

3 Drugs for eradication of *Helicobacter pylori*
- Omeprazole and amoxycillin
- Omeprazole and clarithromycin
- Omeprazole, metronidazole, and clarithromycin/amoxycillin
- Bismuth sub-citrate, etronidazole and tetracycline/amoxycillin

4 H2 receptor antagonists
- Cimetidine
- Famotidine
- Nizatidine
- Ranitidine

5 Mucosal protective agents

  a **Colloid bismuth compounds**
  - Bismuth subcitrate

  b **Liquorice derivatives**
  - Carbenoxolone

  c **Prostaglandin analogue**
  - Misoprostol

  d **Sulphated sucrose complex**
  - Sucralfate

6 Proton pump inhibitors (PPIs)
- Esomeprazole
- Lansoprazole
- Omeprazole
- Pantoprazole

7 Miscellaneous
- Metoclopramide
- Oxethezaine
- Proglumide
- Simethicone

Antipsychotic drugs
A Typical/classical antipsychotics
  1 Phenothiazine derivatives
    a Aliphatic compounds
- Promazine
- Chlorpromazine

    b Piperazine compounds
- Perphenazine
- Fluphenazine

    c Piperidine compounds
- Thioridazine
- Mesoridazine

  2 Butyrophenone derivatives
- Droperidol
- Haloperidol

  3 Thioxanthene derivatives
- Thiothixene
- Flupenthixol

  4 Rauwolfia alkaloids
- Reserpine

B Atypical/newer antipsychotics
- Aripiprazole
- Clozapine
- Olanzapine
- Quetiapine
- Loxapine
- Risperidone
- Ziprasidone

C Drugs used to treat manic-depressive disorders
- Carbamazepine
- Valproic acid
- Lamotrigine
- Lithium carbonate

Antithyroid drugs
1 Thioamides
- Propyl thiouracil
- Methyl thiouracil
- Carbimazole
- Methimazole

2 Anion inhibitors
- Potassium perchlorate

- Thiocyanate
3 Iodides
- Lugol's iodine
- Potassium iodide
4 Radio-active iodine
- I^{131}
5 β-adrenoceptor blockers
- Nadolol
- Propranolol

Beta-blocking drugs
A According to duration of action
  1 Intermediate acting
- Domolol
- Metoprolol
- Pindolol
- Propranolol

  2 Long acting
- Atenolol
- Bisoprolol
- Nadolol

  3 Ultrashort acting
- Esmolol

B According to β receptor selectivity
  1 Both α and β blockers
- Carvedilol
- Labetalol

  2 β1 blocker with partial β2 agonist activity
- Celiprolol

  3 β2 selective blocker
- Butoxamine

  4 Cardioselective (β1) blockers
    i Pure blockers
- Atenolol
- Bisoprolol

    ii With intrinsic sympathetic activity (ISA)
- Practalol

    iii With membrane stabilising activity (MSA)
- Betaxolol
- Metoprolol
- Tolamolol

    iv With both ISA and MSA
- Acebutolol

  5 Non-selective (β1 and β2) blockers
    i Pure blockers
- Nadolol
- Sotalol
- Timolol

  ii **With ISA**
- Carteolol
- Penbutolol

  iii **With MSA**
- Propranolol

  iv **With ISA and MSA**
- Alprenolol
- Pindolol
- Oxprenolol

C According to solubility

 1 Lipid-soluble
- Metoprolol
- Propranolol
- Timolol

 2 Water-soluble
- Atenolol
- Nadolol

Cathartics/drastics/laxatives/purgatives

A According to mechanism of action (MOA)

 1 Stimulant/irritant purgatives

  a **Small gut**
- Castor oil
- Resins

  b **Large gut**
- Bisacodyl
- Anthracene

 2 Bulk-forming purgatives

  a **Colloidal**
- Agar-agar
- Bran
- Calcium polycarbophil
- Frangula
- Isphagol husk
- Methyl-cellulose
- Malt soup extract
- Psyllium husk
- Sterculia

  b **Osmotic**
- Glycerin
- Lactose
- Mannitol
- Sorbitol
- Saline purgatives (e.g. Mg-citrate, $MgCO_3$, MgO, $Mg(OH)_2$, $MgSO_4$, Na_2SO_4, Na^+/K^+ tartarate, Na^+ phosphate)

 3 Fecal softeners
- Docusate Na^+
- Lubricants (arachis oil, liquid paraffin)

4 Miscellaneous
- Calomel
- Colocynth
- Croton oil
- Opioid receptor antagonist
- Parasympathomimetics
- Sulphur
- 5-HT4 receptor agonist

B According to site of action

1 Small intestine
- Castor oil
- Irritant resins

2 Large intestine
- Anthracene derivatives
- Bisacodyl
- Phenolphthalein

3 Small and large intestines
- Lubricants
- Saline purgatives

Parasympathomimetics/cholinomimetics/cholinergic drugs

A Directly acting cholinergic drugs

1 Choline esters
- Acetylcholine
- Methacholine
- Bethanechol
- Carbachol

2 Cholinomimetic alkaloids

a Mainly muscarinic agonists

i Natural alkaloids
- Arecholine
- Muscarine
- Pilocarpine

ii Synthetic alkaloids
- Oxotremorine

b Mainly nicotinic agonists

i Natural alkaloids
- Lobeline
- Nicotine

ii Synthetic alkaloids
- Dimethylphenyl-piperazinium (DMPP)

B Indirectly acting cholinergic drugs

1 Reversible

a Alcohols
- Endrophonium

b Carbamates

i Tertiary amines
- Physostigmine

      ii **Quartenary ammonium compounds**
- Ambenonium
- Demecarium
- Distigmine
- Neostigmine
- Pyridostigmine

  c **Miscellaneous**
- Donepezil
- Galantamine
- Rivastigmine
- Tacrine

2 **Irreversible**

  a **Therapeutically useful**
- Echothiophate

  b **War gases**
- Soman
- Sarin
- Tuban

  c **Insecticides**
- Malathion
- Parathion
- Diisopropyl-fluorophosphate (DFP)
- Octamethyl-pyrophosphotetra-amide (OMPA)
- Tetraethyl-pyrophosphate (TEPP)

Diuretics
A According to mechanism of action (MOA)

1 **Drugs increasing GFR/secondary diuretics**
- Aminophylline
- Caffeine
- Theophylline
- Xanthine

2 **Drugs interfering with ionic transport**

  i **Drugs interfering with ionic transport of bicarbonate (HCO_3)**
- **Carbonic anhydrase inhibitors**
  - Acetazolamide
  - Dichlorphenamide
  - Methazolamide

  ii **Inhibitors of active transport of chloride**

    a **Loop diuretics (high ceiling diuretics)**
- **Carboxylic acid derivatives**
  - Bumetanide
  - Furosemide
  - Piretanide
  - Torsemide
- **Phenoxy-acetic acid derivatives**
  - Ethacrynic acid
  - Indacrinone

    b **Thiazide diuretics**
- Bendrofluazide
- Chlorothiazide
- Hydrochlorothiazide
- Hydroflumethiazide
- Methyl clothiazide
- **Thiazide-related compounds**
- Chlorthalidone
- Indapamide

    iii **Potassium-sparing diuretics**
- **Aldosterone antagonists/receptor blockers**
  - Eplerenone
  - Spironolactone
- **Non-aldosterone antagonists**
  - Amiloride
  - Triamterene

3 **Osmotic diuretics**
- Glycerin
- Isosorbide
- Mannitol
- Urea

B **According to site of action:**
1 **Drugs acting on cortical collecting tubule (CCT)**
- **Potassium-sparing diuretics**
  - Aldosterone antagonists
  - Non-aldosterone antagonists
- **Antidiuretic hormone (ADH) antagonists**
2 **Drugs acting on distal convoluted tubule (DCT)**
- Thiazide diuretics
3 **Drugs acting on proximal convoluted tubule (PCT)**
- Acidifying salts
- Carbonic Anhydrase Inhibitors
- Osmotic diuretics
- Xanthine diuretics
4 **Drugs acting on thick ascending limb (TAL) of Loop of Henle**
- Loop diuretics

Drugs used in diabetes mellitus
A **Insulin**
1 **Intermediate-acting insulins**
- NPH (neutral protamine hagedorn) humulin or novolin insulin; isophane insulin suspension USP
2 **Long-acting insulins**
- Insulin detemir
- Insulin glargine
3 **Pre-mixed insulins**
- Humulin 70/30 and 50/50
- Novolin 70/30

- 70/30 NPA, aspart
- 50/50 NPL, lispro

4 Rapid-acting insulins
- Insulin aspart
- Insulin dlulisine
- Insulin lispro
- Insulin recombinant inhaled

5 Short-acting insulins
- Regular exubera
- Regular humulin or novolin insulin
- Velosulin

B Oral antidiabetic agents

1 Alpha-glucosidase inhibitors
- Acarbose
- Miglitol

2 Biguanides
- Buformin
- Metformin

3 Insulin secretagogues

a D-Phenylalanine derivatives
- Nateglinide

b Meglitinides
- Repaglinide

c Sulfonylureas

i 1st Generation
- Acetohexamide
- Chlorpropamide
- Tolazamide
- Tolbutamide

ii 2nd Generation
- Glibenclamide
- Glimepiride
- Glipizide
- Glyburide

4 Thiazolidinediones
- Pioglitazone
- Rosiglitazone

Drugs used in hyperlipidemia

1 Bile acid binding resins
- Colestipol
- Cholestyramine

2 Competitive inhibitors of HMG-COA reductase
- Fluvastatin
- Lovastatin
- Pravastatin
- Simvastatin

3 Fibric acid derivatives
- Bezafibrate
- Fenofibrate
- Gemfibrozil

4 Inhibitors of intestinal sterol absorption
- Ezetimibe

5 Niacin (nicotinic acid)

H1-receptor antagonists (antihistaminics)

A First generation

1 Alkylamines
- Chlorpheniramine maleate
- Pheniramine maleate
- Triprolidine HCl

2 Ethanolamines
- Clemastine fumarate
- Dimenhydrinate
- Diphenhydramine HCl

3 Ethylene diamines
- Antazoline HCl
- Methapyrilene HCl
- Mepyramine maleate
- Tripelennamine citrate

4 Piperazines
- Buclizine
- Cyclizine HCl
- Chlorcyclizine HCl
- Hydroxyzine HCl
- Meclizine HCl.

5 Phenothiazines
- Dimethothiazine mesylate
- Methdilazine HCl
- Promethazine theoclate
- Trimeprazine tartarate

6 Piperidines
- Astemizole
- Cyproheptadine hydrochloride
- Phenindamine tartarate
- Terfenadine

7 Miscellaneous
- Doxepine hydrochloride
- Mebhydrolin napadisylate

B Second generation

1 Alkylamines (acrivastine)

2 Piperazines (cetrizine hydrochloride)

3 Piperidines (fexofenadine, loratadine)

General anaesthetics
I Inhalational GA
  A Volatile liquids
    1 Older GA
      - Ether
      - Chloroform
    2 Halogenated GA
      - Halothane
      - Isoflurane
      - Methoxyflurane
      - Enflurane
      - Desflurane
      - Sevoflurane
  B Gases
    - Nitrous oxide
    - Xenon
    - Cyclopropane
II Intravenous GA
  1 Barbiturates
    - Thiopentone sodium
    - Hexobarbitone
    - Methohexitone
  2 Non-barbiturates
    a Phencyclidine
      - Ketamine
    b Benzodiazepines
      - Diazepam
      - Lorazepam
      - Midazolam
  3 Neuroleptic analgesia/anaesthesia
    - Fentanyl
    - Droperidol
  4 Opioid analgesics
    - Morphine
    - Alfentanil
    - Remifentanil
    - Sufentanil
  5 Miscellaneous drugs
    - Propofol
    - Etomidate

Local anaesthetics
  1 According to duration of action
    a Short DOA
      - Procaine
    b Medium DOA
      - Cocaine
      - Lidocaine

- Mepivacaine
- Prilocaine

c **Long DOA**
  - Tetracaine
  - Bupivacaine
  - Etidocaine
  - Ropivacaine

2 According to chemistry
  a **Esters**
  - Cocaine
  - Procaine
  - Tetracaine
  - Benzocaine

  b **Amides**
  - Bupivacaine
  - Etidocaine
  - Lidocaine
  - Mepivacaine
  - Prilocaine
  - Ropivacaine

  c **Ethers**
  - Pramoxine

  d **Ketones**
  - Dyclonine

  e **Phenetidin derivatives**
  - Phenacaine

Narcotic (opioid) analgesics

A Based on source

1 Naturally occurring opium alkaloids
  - Morphine
  - Codeine

2 Semi-synthetic derivatives of opium alkaloids
  - Diamorphine (heroin)
  - Etorphine
  - Hydromorphone
  - Oxymorphone
  - Hydrocodone
  - Oxycodone

3 Synthetic morphine substitutes
  a **Pethidine and its congeners**
  - Fentanyl
  - Sufentanil
  - Alfentanil
  - Diphenoxylate
  - Loperamide

  b **Methadone and its congeners**
  - D-propoxyphene

    c **Morphinan compounds**
- Levorphanol

    d **Benzomorphan compounds**
- Pentazocine
- Cyclazocine
- Phenazocine

B Based on agonist-antagonist activities
  i Pure agonists
- Morphine
- Codeine
- Heroin
- Etorphine
- Fentanyl
- Pethidine

  ii Pure antagonists
- Naloxone
- Nalmefene
- Naltrexone

  iii Mixed agonists-antagonists
- Pentazocine
- Cyclazocine
- Meptazinol
- Nalorphine

Penicillins

A Natural penicillins (narrow-spectrum, β-lactamase susceptible penicillins)
- Benzylpenicillin (penicillin 'G')
- Phenoxymethylpenicillin (penicillin 'V')

B Semi-synthetic penicillins
  1 Very narrow-spectrum, β-lactamase resistant penicillins
- Methicillin
- Nafcillin
- Oxacillin
- Dicloxacillin
- Flucloxacillin

  2 Extended spectrum, β-lactamase susceptible penicillins
    a **Aminopenicillins**
- Ampicillin
- Ampicillin pro-drugs (bacampicillin, pivampicillin, talampicillin)
- Amoxycillin alone, and with clavulanate (i.e. augmentin)
- Amoxycillin + flucloxacillin = magnapam

    b **Amidinopenicillins**
- Mecillinam
- Pivmecillinam

    c **Carboxypenicillins**
- Carbenicillin
- Ticarcillin

    d **Ureidopenicillins**
- Azlocillin
- Mezlocillin
- Piperacillin

3 **Other β-lactam drugs**
- Monobactam (aztreonam)
- Carbapenems (imipenem and meropenem)

4 **β-lactamase inhibitors**
- Sulbactam
- Tazobactam
- Sodium or potassium clavulanate

Quinolones

1st Generation
- Cinoxacin
- Nalidixic acid
- Oxolinic acid

2nd Generation

A **Agents with least activity against Gram –ve and Gram +ve bacteria**
- Norfloxacin

B **Agents with excellent activity against Gram –ve and moderate to good activity against Gram +ve bacteria**
- Enoxacin
- Pefloxacin
- Ciprofloxacin
- Lenfloxacin
- Lomefloxacin
- Ofloxacin

C **Agents with excellent activity against Gram –ve and improved activity against Gram +ve bacteria**
- Gatifloxacin
- Moxyfloxacin
- Sparfloxacin
- Trovafloxacin

D **Agents with additional activity against anaerobic bacteria**
- Moxyfloxacin
- Trovafloxacin

Sedative-hypnotics (according to DOA)

A **Barbiturates**
  i **Long-acting**
- Barbitone
- Methyl phenobarbitone
- Phenobarbitone

  ii **Intermediate-acting**
- Amylobarbitone
- Butobarbitone

- Cyclobarbitone
- Pentobarbitone

iii Short-acting
- Quinalbarbitone

iv Ultrashort-acting
- Methohexitone
- Thiopentone sodium

B Benzodiazepines

i Long-acting
- Chlorazepate
- Diazepam
- Flurazepam
- Nitrazepam

ii Intermediate-acting
- Alprazolam
- Estazolam
- Lorazepam
- Oxazepam

iii Short-acting
- Lormetazepam
- Triazolam

C Newer agents

i Imidazopyridine derivatives
- Zaleplon
- Zolpidem

ii 5-HT1A partial agonists
- Buspirone
- Gepirone
- Ipsapirone

D Older agents
- Chloralhydrate
- Glutethemide
- Meprobamate
- Paraldehyde

Skeletal muscle relaxants

A Centrally-acting muscle relaxants

1 Benzodiazepines
- Clorazepate
- Diazepam
- Ketazolam
- Medazepam

2 Benzoxazole derivatives
- Benzimidazole
- Chlorzoxazone
- Zoxazolamine

3 GABA analogue
- Baclofen

4 **Miscellaneous compounds**
- Cyclobenzaprine
- Chlormezanone
- Chlorphensin
- Methocarbamol
- Orphenadrine HCl
- Orphendrine citrate

5 **Propanediol derivatives**
- Carisoprodol
- Mephenesin
- Meprobamate
- Styramate

B **Directly-acting muscle relaxants**
- Dantrolene

C **Neuromuscular blocking agents**

  i **Competitive blocking/nondepolarising agents**
- Alcuronium
- Atracurium
- Dimethyl tubocurarine
- Fazadinium
- Gallamine
- Pancuronium
- Tubocurarine
- Vecuronium

  ii **Depolarising agents**
- Decamethonium
- Suxamethonium
- Suxemethonium

Sulfonamides

1 **Short-acting (well absorbed by mouth and rapidly eliminated)**

  a **General purpose**
- Sulfadiazine
- Sulfadimidine
- Sulfamethoxazole

  b **Mainly for UTI**
- Sulfamethizole
- Sulfisoxazole

2 **Long acting (well absorbed by GIT and slowly eliminated)**
- Sulfadoxine
- Sulfametopyrazine
- Sulfamethoxypyridazine
- Sulfaphenazole

3 **Poorly absorbed by GIT**
- Sulfaguanidine
- Sulfathalidine
- Succinyl Sulfathiazole

4 For topical application
- Sulfacetamide
- Silver Sulfadiazine

5 Miscellaneous group
- Sulfapyridine
- Sulfasalazine

6 Sulfonamide combinations
- Co-trimoxazole (sulfamethoxazole + trimethoprim)
- Fansidar (sulfadoxine + pyrimethamine)

Tetracyclines

1 Based on source

a Natural
- Chlortetracycline
- Oxytetracycline
- Demeclocycline

b Semi-synthetic
- Clomocycline
- Doxycycline
- Lymecycline
- Minocycline
- Methacycline
- Tetracycline

2 Based on duration of action

a Short-acting
- Tetracycline
- Chlortetracycline
- Oxytetracycline
- Clomocycline

b Intermediate-acting
- Methacycline
- Lymecycline
- Demeclocycline

c Long-acting
- Doxycycline
- Minocycline

Thiazide diuretics

1 Intermediate-acting
- Cyclothiazide
- Methylclothiazide
- Quinethazone
- Trichlormethiazide

2 Short-acting
- Bendroflumethiazide
- Cyclopenthiazide
- Chlorothiazide
- Hydrochlorothiazide

- Hydroflumethiazide
3 Long-acting
- Chlorthalidone
- Indapamide
- Polythiazide

Loop diuretics
1 Carboxylic acid derivatives
- Bumetanide
- Furosemide
- Piretanide
- Torsemide

2 Phenoxy acetic acid derivatives
- Ethacrynic Acid
- Indacrinone

Antitussives
A Drugs for productive cough
  1 Expectorants
    a Sedative expectorants
      i Alkaline expectorants
- Potassium acetate and citrate

      ii Nauseant expectorants
- Ammonium carbonate and chloride
- Tincture ipecacuanha

      iii Saline expectorants
- Sodium and potassium iodide

    b Stimulant (aromatic) expectorants
- Creosote
- Guaiacol
- Guaiphenesin
- Terpenehydrate

  2 Mucolytics
- Ambroxol
- Acetylcysteine
- Bromohexine
- Carbocysteine
- Methylcysteine
- Proteolytic enzymes (e.g. pancreatic domase and trypsin)

B Drugs for unproductive cough
  1 Peripheral antitussives
    a Drugs with local anaesthetic activity
- Benzonatate

    b Demulcents
- Liquorice lozenges

    c Steam inhalation
- With tincture menthol

2 **Central antitussives**
  a **Opioid antitussives**
    i **Addicting drugs**
- Dihydromorphinone
- Methadone
- Morphine

    ii **Non-addicting drugs**
- Dihydrocodeinone
- Pholcodine

  b **Non-opioid antitussives**
- Benzonatate
- Carbetapentane
- Chlorphedianol
- Dextromethorphan
- Narcotine
- Oxeladine

Drugs used in cardiac failure

1 ACE inhibitors
- Captopril
- Enalapril
- Lisinopril

2 Cardiotonic drugs
  i **β1-selective adrenoceptor agonists**
- Dobutamine
- Prenalterol

  ii **Bipyridine derivatives**
- Inamrinone
- Milrinone

  iii **Cardiac glycosides**
- Digoxin
- Digitoxin
- Gitoxin
- Gitaloxin
- Ouabain
- Strophanthin

3 Diuretics
  i **Loop diuretics**
- Ethacrynic acid
- Furosemide

  ii **Thiazide diuretics**
- Bendrofluazide
- Polythiazide

4 Vasodilators
- Hydralazine
- Nifedipine
- Nitroglycerin
- Prazosin

- Sodium nitroprusside

Therapeutic classification of anti-epileptic drugs

A Drugs used in partial (focal) epilepsy

1 **For simple partial epilepsy**
   - Lamotrigine
   - Felbamate
   - Phenytoin
   - Carbamazepine
   - Primidone
   - Gabapentin
   - Vigabatrin
   - Topiramate

2 **For complex partial/psychomotor/temporal-lobe epilepsy and Jacksonian epilepsy**
   - Phenytoin
   - Carbamazepine
   - Primidone
   - Gabapentin
   - Vigabatrin
   - Topiramate

B Drugs used in generalised epilepsy

1 **For grand-mal epilepsy/generalised tonic-clonic seizures**
   - Sodium valproate
   - Phenobarbitone
   - Primidone
   - Gabapentin
   - Vigabatrin
   - Lamotrigine
   - Felbamate

2 **Petit-mal epilepsy/absence seizures**
   - Sodium valproate
   - Clonazepam
   - Ethosuximide

3 **Atonic seizures**
   - Sodium valproate
   - Clonazepam
   - Nitrazepam

4 **Myoclonic seizures**
   - Clonazepam

5 **Febrile seizures (in children)**
   - Phenobarbitone
   - Primidone

6 **Infantile spasms**
   - Corticotropin
   - Vigabatrin
   - Nitrazepam

7 **Status epilepticus**
- Diazepam
- Fosphenytoin
- Thiopentone sodium
- Phenobarbitone

Therapeutic classification of benzodiazepines
1 **Sedative/hypnotics**
- Flurazepam
- Nitrazepam
- Triazolam
- Lormetazepam

2 **Anxiolytics**
- Diazepam
- Lormetazepam
- Oxazepam

3 **Anticonvulsants**
- Diazepam
- Clonazepam
- Nitrazepam

4 **Central muscle relaxants**
- Diazepam
- Clonazepam
- Flurazepam

3

Mechanisms of action

Reversible anticholinesterases

Drugs included: neostigmine, physostigmine, edrophonium and echothiophate.

Acetylcholine released in the synaptic cleft is degraded into acetate and choline by an enzyme acetylcholinesterase thus terminating its action. This enzyme is found bound to both pre- and postsynaptic membranes. Anticholinesterases inhibit this enzyme thus blocking acetylcholine degradation and prolonging its action. These drugs stimulate all acetylcholine receptors in the body, i.e. muscarinic and nicotinic receptors of ANS, nicotinic receptors present at NMJ and CNS cholinoceptors.

1 *Physostigmine*: It is a reversible anticholinesterase. Chemically it is a carbamic acid ester and a substrate for acetylcholinesterase. The action of acetylcholinesterase on this drug results in the formation of a relatively stable *carbamoylated intermediate with the enzyme*, which thus becomes inactive. This in turn leads to prolongation of acetylcholine action on cholinoceptors throughout the body. The duration of action of physostigmine is about 2–4 hours.

2 *Donezepil, Rivastigmine and Galantamine*: These drugs are also reversible anticholinesterases and are primarily used in the treatment of Alzheimer's disease. The basic pathology in Alzheimer's disease is a deficiency of cholinergic neurons in the CNS. By inhibiting acetylcholinesterase enzyme and thus acetylcholine degradation these drugs try to overcome the deficiency of cholinergic neurons in the brain. Studies have shown that these drugs do slow the progression of Alzheimer's disease, but only for a time being. The main side effect of these drugs is GI upset.

Irreversible anticholinesterases

Drugs included: It includes organophosphate compounds like isoflurophate, parathion, etc.

Chemically these drugs are organophosphorous compounds. Their mechanism of action is similar to other anticholinesterases; the only difference is that these agents covalently bind to acetylcholinesterase, thus permanently and irreversibly inactivating it so that reactivation of acetylcholinesterase activity requires the synthesis of new enzyme molecules. The net result is a long-lasting increase in the cholinergic activity throughout the body (↑ lacrimation, salivation, sweating, miosis, NVD, etc.), motor paralysis (→ breathing difficulty) and convulsions. Owing to such toxic effects these drugs have been developed for military use as nerve agents. The prototype amongst these is isoflurophate.

Isoflurophate: This organophosphorous compound covalently binds with the enzyme anticholinesterase thus inhibiting it permanently. Anticholinesterase activity is restored only once new enzyme molecules are synthesised by the body.

Acetylcholinesterase reactivators (pralidoxime): Since the human body on its own cannot cleave the covalent bond between anticholinesterase enzyme and isoflurophate, the enzyme inactivation is permanent. However, scientists have developed chemical reactivators such as pralidoxime, which, if given within the first few hours of nerve agent exposure, can cleave this covalent bond, thus causing anticholinesterase reactivation and correction of muscle paralysis, breathing difficulties and convulsions. The only shortfall of anticholinesterase reactivators is that these agents are effective only before 'aging' has occurred. 'Aging' refers to the phenomenon of release of one of the alkyl groups by the anticholinesterase-isoflurophate moiety. Once an alkyl group is lost (i.e. aging has occurred), even chemical reactivators like pralidoxime also become ineffective, i.e. they can no longer cleave the covalent bond between anticholinesterase and isoflurophate. Isoflurophate ages in 6–8 hours. Thus, to be effective, it is necessary that pralidoxime is given within this period. The newer nerve agents, available to the military, age within minutes or even seconds.

Antidote of irreversible anticholinesterases: Atropine, by inhibiting antimuscarinic receptors, acts as an antidote of irreversible anticholinesterases. Until the body synthesises new molecules of anticholinesterase enzyme, we can use atropine (in high doses) to block many of the muscarinic and central effects of isoflurophate.

Castor oil

It is a stimulant laxative. In the small intestine, it is broken down to ricinoleic acid, which increases intestinal peristaltic activity, thus relieving constipation. Exaggerated peristaltic activity can produce abdominal cramps. Protracted use of stimulant laxatives is not advisable as they can cause atonic colon with prolonged use.

Cascata, senna and aloe are other agents, which are used as laxatives. These contain emodin – the principal agent that stimulates colonic peristaltic activity. These agents are first absorbed in the small intestine and later excreted into the colon. The onset of action of these agents is thus delayed by 6–8 hours. This delay is, in fact, beneficial because one tablet of senna taken at bedtime causes bowel movement not before early in the morning.

Regulation of gastric HCl secretion

Gastric HCl is produced and secreted by parietal cells. Acetylcholine, histamine and gastrin stimulate parietal cells whereas prostaglandin E_2 and somatostatin inhibit them. Parietal cells have membrane receptors for all these agents.

When stimulants attach with their respective receptors, there occurs activation of protein kinases. Histamine initially causes activation of adenylyl cyclase enzyme, which in turn causes activation of protein kinases. Acetylcholine and gastrin, however, cause Ca^{++} influx. This in turn causes a rise in intracellular Ca^{++} levels and activation of protein kinases. Protein kinases in turn activate the H^+/K^+-ATPase proton pump. This pump actively secretes one H^+ ion into the gastric lumen in exchange for one K^+ ion pumped into the parietal cell from gastric lumen. Additionally, one Cl^- ion is secreted from the parietal cell into the gastric lumen via a separate Cl^- channel. Within the gastric lumen H^+ and Cl^- join to form HCl.

When inhibitors like prostaglandin E_2 bind with their respective receptors, there occurs inactivation of adenylyl cyclase enzyme. This in turn causes inactivation of protein kinases and H^+/K^+-ATPase proton pump thus inhibiting HCl formation.

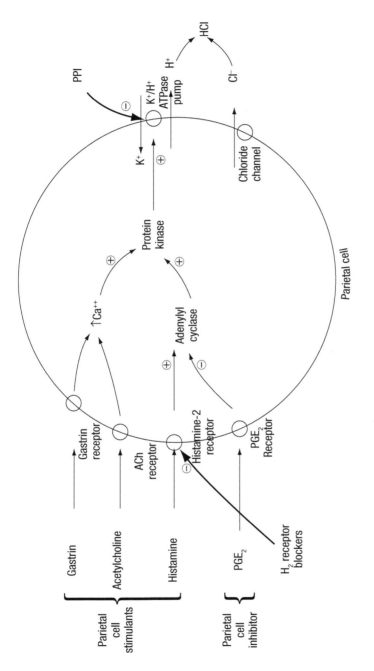

Figure 3.1 Regulation of gastric HCl secretion in parietal cells

Proton Pump Inhibitors (PPIs): These drugs are given orally in the form of capsules in which enteric-coated granules are enclosed to protect them from HCl destruction in the stomach. In intestines, shell is dissolved and granules are liberated. They are highly lipid-soluble and absorbed completely and rapidly from the intestines. Through blood, they reach their site of action, i.e. gastric canaliculi lined by parietal cells. Since the fluid in the gastric canaliculi is acidic and PPIs are basic in nature, the latter get ionised/protonated and trapped in the canaliculi, leading to a 1000-fold rise in their concentration. They are pro-drugs. They are activated into sulfenamide and sulfenic acid, which are interconvertible. These inhibitors combine with H^+/K^+-ATPase proton pump (via the SH-group of cysteine amino acids in the extracellular domain of the proton pump) thus inhibiting it. This leads to total inhibition of HCl synthesis (called anacidity).

Antacids: Antacids are weak bases that react with gastric HCl to form salt and water. Although their principal mechanism of action is reduction of intragastric acidity, they may also promote mucosal defence mechanisms through stimulation of mucosal prostaglandin production. After a meal approximately 45 mEq/hr of HCl is secreted. A single dose of 156 mEq of antacid given 01 hr after a meal effectively neutralises gastric acid for up to 01 hr. However, acid neutralisation capacity among different proprietary formulations of antacids is highly variable depending on their:

1 Rate of dissolution (tablet vs liquid).
2 Water solubility.
3 Rate of reaction with acid.
4 Rate of gastric emptying.

Antileukotriene drugs

Drugs included: zileuton; zafirlukast; montelukast.

Leukotrienes are one of the many pro-inflammatory mediators released by the mast cells (and many other cells including basophils, eosinophils and neutrophils). The 5-lipoxygenase pathway of arachidonic acid metabolism leads to the formation of leukotrienes B_4 (LTB_4) and cysteinyl leukotrienes (which include LTC_4, LTD_4 and LTE_4). Physiologically, LTB_4 is a powerful chemoattractant for neutrophils and eosinophils. Cysteinyl leukotrienes, on the other hand, cause bronchoconstriction and increased endothelial permeability ($\rightarrow \uparrow$ mucus secretion). The net result is narrowing of the airways. Antileukotriene drugs block the leukotriene-induced narrowing of the airways.

Zileuton directly inhibits the 5-lipoxygenase enzyme, thus blocking the synthesis of all leukotrienes. Zafirlukast and montelukast, on the other hand, reversibly inhibit the cysteinyl leukotriene-1 receptor, thus blocking the cysteinyl leukotrienes from exerting their physiological actions.

Antileukotriene drugs are only approved for asthma prophylaxis. In cases of acute, severe, attack of asthma in which immediate bronchodilatation is required, these drugs are not very effective (β_2-agonists like salbutamol, terbutaline, and anticholinergic drugs like ipratropium bromide are effective in emergency situations). When used as prophylactic agents, these drugs improve the respiratory functions and cause modest reductions in the doses of other antiasthmatics agents like β_2-agonists and corticosteroids.

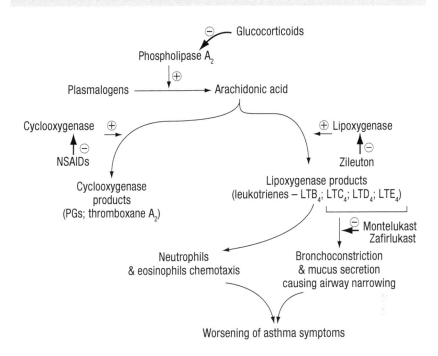

Figure 3.2 **Arachidonic acid metabolism**

Cromolyn and nedocromil

These agents are mast-cell stabilisers. They decrease the release of pro-inflammatory mediators (like histamine and leukotrienes) from the mast cells. They do not in any way block the effects of those mediators that have already been released. Thus the only role of these agents is in asthma prophylaxis. Unlike β_2-agonists, they cannot cause bronchodilatation; they can just prevent bronchoconstriction. They are particularly useful in allergic asthma in children, in whom they prevent allergen-induced bronchoconstriction and thus precipitation of an acute attack of asthma.

These agents are extremely insoluble and thus poorly absorbed so that even large doses of these agents given orally yield sub-therapeutic blood levels. Thus the only way to give these drugs is by aerosols in asthma patients.

Thiazide diuretics

As diuretic: After having reached their site of action at distal-convoluted tubules (DCT), thiazide diuretics inhibit reabsorption of NaCl by inhibiting NaCl symporter or co-transporter. NaCl is excreted by an equal amount of water to cause diuresis. Thiazides are moderate efficacy diuretics – only 5–10% of total Na^+ load in tubular filtrate is inhibited by these drugs.

As antihypertensive:

A Initially there is a transient fall in blood pressure because of the diuretic effect as explained below:

$\uparrow$ Excretion of NaCl $\rightarrow$ $\downarrow$ ECF volume $\rightarrow$ $\downarrow$ venous return and cardiac output $\rightarrow$ $\downarrow$ BP.

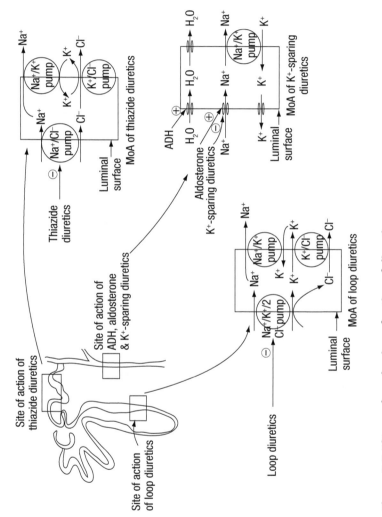

Figure 3.3 Sites and mechanism of action of diuretics.

Once ECF volume is made up by compensatory mechanism in the body (i.e. more NaCl and water reabsorption from DCT), blood pressure returns to normal.

B Natriuretic action: ↓ concentration of Na^+ in vascular beds → loss of response of vascular smooth muscles to circulating catecholamines → vasodilatation → fall in BP.

Good points of thiazide diuretics as an antihypertensive include the following:

A Cost-effectiveness.

B Good compliance.

C Convenient route of administration – oral.

D Antihypertensive/diuretic effect is independent of metabolic acidosis or alkalosis.

E To have synergistic effect, they are combined with other antihypertensive drugs (like ACEIs, beta-blockers).

F Since the therapeutic index is high, these drugs are reasonably safe.

Loop diuretics

Main mechanism: On oral administration, having being absorbed readily, they are secreted in the proximal convoluted tubules (PCT) by an active secretory process, which is specific for organic acids. They reach their site of action, i.e. thick ascending limb (TAL) of loop of Henle. Here they inhibit the $Na^+/K^+/2Cl^-$ transporter, resulting in NaCl reabsorption inhibition from TAL of loop of Henle. NaCl in the urinary filtrate produces osmotic pressure and inhibits reabsorption of water from the remaining parts of nephron. As compared to thiazide diuretics, loop diuretics cause a greater volume of water and solutes to be excreted from the kidneys. Between 15% and 25% of total Na^+ load in tubular filtrate is inhibited by these drugs, leading to massive diuresis.

Contributory mechanisms:

A Decreased filtration fraction (the ratio of GFR/renal blood flow).

B Interference with counter-current multiplier exchange system.

C Changes in renal hemodynamic state.

D Decrease degradation of PGI_2 and PGE_2.

Potassium-sparing diuretics

Potassium-sparing diuretics prevent K^+ secretion by antagonising the effects of aldosterone at the late distal and cortical collecting tubules. Inhibition may occur either by direct pharmacologic antagonism of mineralocorticoid receptors (spironolactone and eplerenone) or by inhibition of Na^+ influx through ion channels in the luminal membrane (amiloride and triamterene).

Sulfonylureas
Effects on pancreas

1 These agents are insulin secretagogues, i.e. they stimulate insulin release from pancreatic β-cells by blocking the ATP-sensitive K^+ channels. They have specific binding receptors on the ATP-sensitive K^+ channels. The ligand-receptor binding leads to decreased K^+ efflux, leading to depolarisation of the β-cells. Also, it causes opening up of the voltage-dependent Ca^{++} channels. Ca^{++} influx in turn causes increased insulin release from the β-cells, leading to lowering of the glucose levels.

2 Decrease in serum glucagon level.

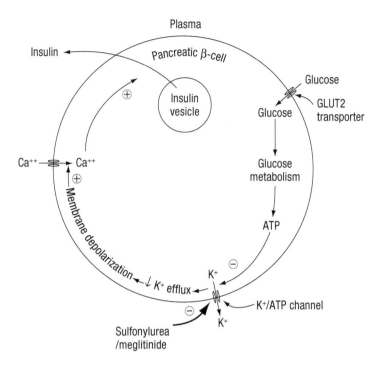

Figure 3.4 **Physiology of insulin release from pancreatic β-cells, and mechanism of action of sulfonylurea and meglitinide**

Effect on peripheral insulin receptors

3 Unregulation of insulin receptors on target organs thus enhancing peripheral utilisation of glucose (especially in muscles and adipose tissue).

Effects on liver

4 Decrease in hepatic insulin degradation.
5 Decrease in hepatic gluconeogenesis.

Note: It is important to understand here that the main pharmacologic effect of sulfonylureas (i.e. ↑ insulin secretion from the pancreas) is dependent on functioning β-cells. In type-1 diabetes mellitus in which β-cells are destroyed (probably by an autoimmune mechanism), these agents are ineffective.

Meglitinides

Just like sulfonylureas, these agents are insulin secretagogues, i.e. they stimulate insulin release from pancreatic β-cells. Their mechanism of action is also similar to that of sulfonylureas, i.e. they block the ATP-sensitive K+ channels (→ ↑ insulin secretion). Meglitinides have two binding sites in common with sulfonylureas and one unique binding site.

The difference between sulfonylureas and meglitinides is that the latter have a rapid onset and short duration of action as compared to the former. Thus they are particularly effective in increasing insulin levels immediately after meals, thus correcting post-prandial hyperglycemia. In order to avoid post-prandial hyperglycemia, these agents are given from 1 to 30 minutes before meals.

An advantage of meglitinides is that these agents lack sulphur in their structure. Thus they can be used in type-2 diabetics with sulphur or sulfonylurea allergy. Also, combination therapy of meglitinides and metformin has been shown to be better than monotherapy with either agent in achieving normoglycemia.

Biguanides
Biguanides produce their pharmacological effects by multiple mechanisms including:
1 Reduced hepatic and renal gluconeogenesis. It is pertinent to mention here that increased glucose output by the liver is the main cause of hyperglycemia in type-2 diabetics.
2 Slowing of glucose absorption from GIT with increase glucose to lactate conversion by enterocytes.
3 Direct stimulation of glycolysis in tissues with increased glucose removal from the blood.
4 Reduction in plasma glucagon levels.
5 Another beneficial effect of these drugs is lowering the levels of 'bad cholesterol' (i.e. LDL and VLDL cholesterol) and rising that of 'good cholesterol' (i.e. HDL cholesterol). These effects become apparent after 4–6 weeks of continuous use.
6 Biguanides cause anorexia → ↓ food intake → ↓ glucose level. These drugs are thus the preferred antidiabetics in overweight/obese diabetics.

Because of the above-mentioned multiple beneficial effects, biguanides are the *only* oral hypoglycemics proven to decrease cardiovascular mortality.

Thiazolidinediones (TZDs)
Effect on insulin resistance: TZDs act by decreasing insulin resistance. Their target receptor is called peroxisome proliferator-activated receptor-gamma (PPAR-γ). These receptors are found in liver, adipose tissue and skeletal muscles. PPAR-γ receptors are complex and modulate expression of genes involved in:
1 Lipid and glucose metabolism.
2 Insulin signal transduction.
3 Adipocyte and other tissue differentiation.
4 Secretion of fatty acids.

The net effect of PPAR-γ receptors stimulation is increased insulin sensitivity (or decreased insulin resistance) in liver, adipose tissue and skeletal muscles.

Since the mechanism of action of TZDs involves gene regulation, they have slow onset and offset of activity over weeks or even months.

Effects on adipose tissue and lipid levels
1 In adipose tissue the drug promotes glucose uptake and utilisation.
2 Both pioglitazone and rosiglitazone increase the level of good cholesterol (i.e. HDL cholesterol). The level of bad cholesterol (i.e. LDL cholesterol) is lowered

by pioglitazone but raised by rosiglitazone. Besides this, another bad effect of rosiglitazone is that this drug causes oedema, especially when combined with insulin. Rosiglitazone-insulin combination is thus not recommended.

3 TZDs regulate adipocyte apoptosis and differentiation in such a way that there occurs an expansion in the subcutaneous fat.

TZDs also have significant effects on vascular endothelium, immune system, ovaries and tumour cells.

α-glucosidase inhibitors
Drugs included: acarbose; miglitol.

α-glucosidase inhibitors are competitive inhibitors of membrane-bound α-glucosidases (sucrase, maltase, glycoamylase, dextranase) in the intestinal brush border. α-glucosidases cause hydrolysis of oligosaccharides to glucose and other sugars. By inhibiting this enzyme, these drugs delay the digestion and thus absorption of ingested starch and disaccharides thus avoiding postprandial hyperglycemia. In fact post-prandial glycemic excursions are lowered by as much as 45–60 mg/dl. Thus the need of increased post-prandial release of insulin to control postprandial hyperglycemia is lowered by these drugs – an insulin-sparing effect.

Differences b/w acarbose and miglitol:

1 *Difference in potency*: Miglitol differs structurally as well as in binding affinity from acarbose and is six times more potent in inhibiting sucrase.

2 *Difference in α-glucosidases targeted*: Miglitol alone inhibits isomaltase and β-glucosidases, which split β-linked sugars such as lactose. Similarly, acarbose alone inhibits α-amylase.

Colchicine
Colchicine primarily produces its anti-inflammatory effects by binding to an intracellular microtubular protein called tubulin in granulocytes and other motile cells causing its depolymerisation. This in turn causes inhibition of leukocyte migration to the site of inflammation ($\rightarrow \downarrow$ phagocytosis at the site of inflammation).

Other anti-inflammatory effects include:

A Decreased release of inflammatory mediators responsible for pain (e.g. lactic acid and lipoproteins). Colchicine is in fact known to alleviate the pain of acute gout within 12 hours.

B Inhibition of synthesis and release of proinflammatory mediators (e.g. prostaglandins and leukotriene B4).

C Blockage of cellular division by binding to mitotic spindles.

Allopurinol
After oral administration, allopurinol is approximately 80% absorbed and has a terminal serum t½ of 1–2hrs. Allopurinol inhibits uric acid synthesis:

Hypoxanthine → xanthine → uric acid

Xanthine oxidase is the catalysing enzyme for both these steps.

Allopurinol is a pro-drug. It is metabolised by xanthine oxidase enzyme to alloxanthine. Alloxanthine in turn inhibits xanthine oxidase enzyme thus inhibiting uric acid synthesis and increasing the concentrations of hypoxanthine and xanthine. Alloxanthine has a long duration of action so that allopurinol needs to be given only once daily.

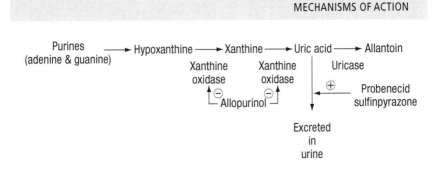

Figure 3.5 **Purine metabolism and pharmacological interventions with allopurinol, probenecid and sulfinpyrazone**

Morphine

Opioid receptors are present both in the ascending pathways responsible for pain *transmission* from the periphery to the higher centres and the descending pathways (in midbrain and medulla) responsible for pain *modulation*.

Action at post-synaptic level: agonistic action on Mu (μ) receptors with resultant opening up of K⁺ channels: Morphine binds to specific opioid receptors situated in the GIT, urinary

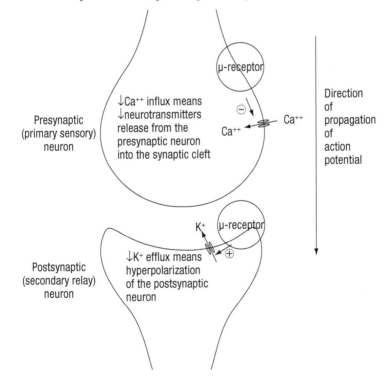

Figure 3.6 **Mechanism of action of morphine (μ-receptor agonists)**

bladder and other smooth muscles as well as in CNS (brain and spinal cord including peri-aqueductal grey matter, nucleus rafimagnus, nucleus reticularis, paragigantocellularis, substantia gelatinosa, limbic system and in somatosensory cortical area). Mu (μ) receptors have got great affinity for morphine. When morphine binds to these receptors, it causes opening up of K^+ channels with resultant efflux of K^+ ions and hyperpolarisation at postsynaptic neurons causing neuronal depression.

Action at pre-synaptic level: agonistic action on mu (μ), kappa (κ) and delta (δ) receptors with resultant closure of pre-synaptic, voltage-gated, Ca++ channels: Morphine acts on μ, κ, δ receptors found on the pre-synaptic terminals of the nociceptive primary afferents resulting in closure of the pre-synaptic, voltage-gated Ca^{++} channels present. Inhibition of Ca^{++} influx inhibits the release of neurotransmitters like acetylcholine, norepinephrine, serotonin, somatostatin, bombesin and substance P. These neurotransmitters mediate pain perception in the spinal cord. When their release into the synaptic cleft is inhibited, post-synaptic neuronal firing and thus transmission of nociception decreases.

Action at the periphery: *Agonistic action on delta (δ) receptors with resultant depression of peripheral nociceptors*: Morphine and other opioid analgesics also depress the discharge from the peripheral nociceptive afferent neurons. This in turn leads to impaired nociceptive input and thus impaired pain perception.

At molecular level, it is pertinent to mention here that all three opioid receptors (μ, κ, δ) are coupled to their effectors by G proteins, and activate phospholipase C or inhibit adenylyl cyclase.

Box 3.1 CNS effects of morphine

1 Analgesia. Both the sensory and emotional aspects of pain experience are attenuated, i.e. although patients are still aware of the presence of pain, the sensation is not unpleasant.

2 Sedation via κ-receptor activation. At higher doses, it can even cause stupor and coma.

3 Euphoria. By stimulating ventral tegmentum, morphine produces a powerful sense of well-being and euphoria.

4 Miosis (except mepridine, which has a muscarinic blocking action). Nalaxone (an opioid antagonist) and atropine can reverse miosis.

5 Inhibition of respiratory centre in medulla oblongata via μ-receptor activation with resultant decreased response to PCO_2 ($\rightarrow \uparrow PCO_2 \rightarrow$ cerebrovascular dilatation $\rightarrow \uparrow$ ICP).

6 Nausea and vomiting (by activating chemoreceptor trigger zone). Anti-emetics are routinely given with morphine and other narcotic analgesic injections.

7 Suppression of cough reflex (by an unknown mechanism).

Benzodiazepines (BDZs)

GABA (γ-aminobutyric acid) is the major inhibitory neurotransmitter in the CNS. Benzodiazepines are GABA-ergic (meaning they potentiate the post-synaptic inhibitory actions of GABA in various areas of the brain). GABA receptors are composed of α, β, and γ-subunits. Five or more combinations of these subunits constitute the different

Pain transmission from nociceptors to cerebral cortex. Since different painkillers act at different/multiple sites, a combination of them is more effective than monotherapy with any one analgesic agent

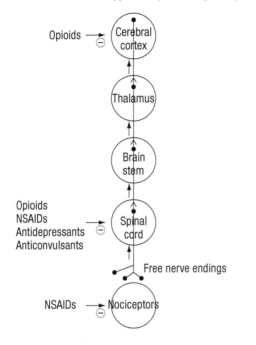

Figure 3.7 Pain transmission from nociceptors to cerebral cortex

GABA receptor subtypes present on the post-synaptic membranes in the CNS. Depending upon the subtype activated, varying pharmacological effects of BDZs are produced (Table 3.1).

BDZs bind with 'BDZ-binding sites' located at the interface of α, and γ_2-subunits. This leads to displacement of a substance GABA-modulin, which occupies GABA receptors and keeps them in a relatively non-functional state. This in turn increases the affinity GABA for its receptor (GABA$_A$) leading to increased opening up of chloride channels, hyper-polarisation and thus depression of the post-synaptic neurons. In other words, BDZs increase the affinity GABA for its receptor, in turn increasing the frequency of chloride channels opening produced by GABA.

It is pertinent to mention here that BDZs are not GABA-mimetic (meaning they do not have effects like GABA) and the presence of GABA in the CNS is necessary for the actions of BDZs. If we inhibit the synthesis of GABA with thiosemicarbazide, BDZs become ineffective. Similarly if we block post-synaptic receptors of GABA with bicuculline, BDZs again will become ineffective.

Table 3.1

Receptor activated	Effects
α_2- GABA$_A$ → Inhibition of neuronal circuits in the limbic system	Reduction in anxiety (anxiolytic effect)
α_2- GABA$_A$ → increased pre-synaptic inhibition in the spinal cord (at higher doses)	Skeletal muscle relaxation
α_1- GABA$_A$	• Hypnosis (artificially produced sleep) • Anterograde amnesia (temporary impairment of memory) • Anticonvulsant effect

BDZs do not affect the autonomic nervous system. Also, they lack any antipsychotic or analgesic activity.

Local anaesthetics

As we know that Na$^+$ influx is necessary for depolarisation to take place. It is also necessary for conduction of the wave of depolarisation. Local anaesthetics, by blocking the voltage-gated Na$^+$ channels, block both generation and conduction of the action potential and in this way produce a membrane-stabilising effect.

Location of receptor sites: Local anaesthetics block the Na$^+$ channels from the cytosolic side. They must, therefore, cross the lipid membrane and diffuse into the cytoplasm before they could reach their receptor sites in the Na$^+$ channel.

Two forms of local anaesthetic molecules: Local anaesthetic molecules are available both in the nonionised (uncharged) and ionised (charged) forms. The nonionised molecules are more lipid-soluble and thus have greater ability to diffuse across the lipid membrane and reach effective intracellular concentrations within the cytoplasm. The ionised molecules, however, have greater affinity for the receptor sites. Thus availability of both the nonionised and ionised forms is important for the functioning of the local anaesthetics.

Effects of ECF K$^+$ and Ca^{++} on local anaesthetic activity:
- ↑ ECF K$^+$ → ↑ local anaesthetic activity.
- ↑ ECF Ca^{++} → ↓ local anaesthetic activity.

Order of loss of sensations: Autonomic sensations are lost first after local anaesthetic injection followed by pain, touch, vibration and deep pressure sensations (in this order) and finally motor activity.

The order of loss of sensations depends on:
1 Diameter of the nerve fibres: Smaller fibres are blocked more easily than the larger fibres.
2 Myelination of the nerve fibres: Myelinated fibres are blocked more easily than the unmyelinated fibres.
3 Physiologic firing rate of the nerve fibres: Rapidly firing fibres are usually blocked before the slowly firing fibres.

Ketamine

Ketamine is a short-acting, non-barbiturate anaesthetic. It characteristically produces 'dissociative anaesthesia' in which patient appears to be awake but is immobile, doesn't feel pain and is amnesic.

Ketamine antagonises the actions of glutamic acid (an excitatory neurotransmitter) on the N-methyl-D-aspartate (NMDA) receptor. It also increases the central sympathetic outflow ($\rightarrow$ bronchodilatation, $\uparrow$ cardiac output and $\uparrow$ BP). Because of this property, Ketamine is especially beneficial in cases of asthma and shock (cardiogenic; hypovolemic). Because of the same property it is not recommended in cases of hypertension and stroke.

Haloperidol

Haloperidol is a typical (traditional) neuroleptic agent used in the treatment of schizophrenia and other psychoses.

Dopamine hypothesis of schizophrenia: It appears that schizophrenia, at least in part, is caused by an excess of dopamine in the mesolimbic pathway of the brain (regulates mood and mentation).

Types of dopamine receptors: Five types of dopamine receptors have been identified (D_1-D_5). D_1 and D_5 receptors activate adenylyl cyclase, whereas, D_2, D_3 and D_4 receptors inhibit adenylyl cyclase.

Table 3.2 Location of dopamine receptors

Location of dopamine receptors	Responsible for	Effect of dopamine receptor blockade
Mesolimbic pathway	Regulates mood and mentation	Antipsychotic effect
Nigrostriatal pathway	Extrapyramidal function	Extrapyramidal symptoms
Tuberoinfundibular pathway	Control of prolactin release	Hyperprolactinemia
Chemoreceptor trigger zone	Emesis	Anti-emetic effect

Receptors affected by haloperidol:
1 Haloperidol exerts its antipsychotic effect by primarily blocking the D_2 receptors present in caudate, putamen, nucleus accumbens, cerebral cortex and hypothalamus.
2 Antipsychotic effect is also in part produced by haloperidol-induced α_1 receptor blockade.
3 Many of the newer atypical antipsychotic agents also block 5-HT_2, H_1 and M receptors. Haloperidol lacks effect on any of these receptors.

Antipsychotic effects of haloperidol: Haloperidol reduces the 'positive' symptoms of schizophrenia;[1] it, however, has little effect on the 'negative' symptoms.[2]

Barbiturates
1 There are multiple mechanisms of action of barbiturates at multiple sites in the brain. They act on $GABA_A$ receptor Cl$^-$ channel.
2 Macromolecular complex.
3 GABA-ergic at low doses, i.e. facilitation of action of GABA and prolongation of Cl$^-$ channels opening.

---

1 Positive symptoms of schizophrenia: hallucinations, delusions.

2 Negative symptoms of schizophrenia: impaired attention, cognitive impairment, apathy, anhedonia (not getting pleasure from normally pleasurable stimuli).

4 GABA-mimetic at high doses, i.e. directly activates Cl⁻ channels.
5 Barbiturates are less sedative in their action since they also depress the actions of excitatory neurotransmitters (NT), e.g. glutamic acid.
6 Actions of excitatory NT, i.e. glutamic acid (at AMP_A receptor subtype) depressed.
7 Potentiation of inhibitory $GABA_A$ receptors.
8 Inhibition of excitatory AMP_A receptors leading to CND depressant effect.
9 Higher concentration inhibits Ca^{++}.

Carbamazepine

1 Carbamazepine blocks voltage-dependent Na^+ channels and inhibits the spread of discharge.
2 Acts pre-synaptically to decrease the synaptic transmission.
3 Post-synaptic actions of GABA may be potentiated.
4 Also inhibits uptake and release of norepinephrine from the brain.

Phenytoin sodium

It is a membrane stabiliser and acts by:
1 Decreasing the resting fluxes of Na^+ ions as well as Na^+ currents during the action potential.
2 Decreasing the influx of Ca^{++} ions during depolarisation.
3 Decreasing the efflux of K^+ ions during action potential.
4 Decrease in post-tetanic potentiation.
5 Restoration of balance between excitatory glutamate and inhibitory GABA pathways.
6 Decrease in the duration of after-discharge.
7 Increase in the refractory period of the neurons.
8 Causes stimulation of cerebellum, which in turn causes stimulation of inhibitory pathways from cerebellum to cerebral cortex.

The above-mentioned processes show that phenytoin sodium causes:
1 A decrease in the development of maximal seizure activity from the epileptic focus.
2 A decrease in the spread of seizure activity from an active focus.

Sodium valproate/valproic acid

GABA, which is the main inhibitory NT in the brain, is synthesised from glutamic acid (glutamate) in GABA-ergic neurons by an enzyme called glutamic acid decarboxylase. GABA is metabolised sequentially by GABA transaminase into succinic-semialdehyde, then into succinic acid by the enzyme succinic-semialdehyde dehydrogenase.

Main mechanism of action of sodium valproic is to raise GABA concentration in the CNS by inhibiting above-mentioned both enzymes responsible for the metabolism of GABA resulting in increased inhibition of neurons in the CNS. Sodium valproic also enhances GABA post-synaptic actions. It has a weak Na^+ channels blocking effect and also causes small decrease in low threshold Ca^{++} channels.

Chlorpromazine (largactil)

It acts on a variety of CNS and peripheral receptors and causes:
1 Post-synaptic dopamine (D_2) receptor blockade.
2 $5HT_{2A}$ and $5HT_{2C}$ serotinergic receptor blockade.

3 Muscarinic and ganglion receptor blockade.
4 α1 adrenoceptor and H1 histaminic receptor blockade.
5 Quinidine and local anaesthetic-like activity.

Effects on CNS

1 *General psycho-physiological and behavioural effects*:
   a Neuroleptic syndrome: characterised by apathy and indifference, suppression of psychomotor and spontaneous activity, decreased hallucinations, decreased illusions, decrease in stereotype behaviour, decrease in incoherent thoughts and suppression of conditioned avoidance behaviour (does not suppress unconditioned responses).
   b Catalepsy: Cataleptic immobility means maintaining of abnormal posture in animals and humans.
   c 5HT receptor blockade leads to disturbances in mood, behaviour and sleep.
2 *Effects on motor activity*: Decreased spontaneous activity, extrapyramidal symptoms (Parkinsonism, acute dystonias, akathesias, tardive dyskinesia, perioral tremors [Rabbit syndrome]).
3 *Effects on chemoreceptor trigger zone* (CTZ): It blocks CTZ in D_2 receptor area in the medulla suppressing nausea and vomiting; hence used as anti-emetic.
4 *Hypothalamic and endocrine effects*: By blocking α-1 receptors ADH, oestrogen, progesterone, corticosteroids and growth hormone levels are decreased.

Peripheral effects

1 *Effects on ANS*: By blocking muscarinic receptors, atropine-like effects are seen, e.g. dryness of mouth, tachycardia, blurring of vision, etc.
2 *Effects on CVS*:
   a α-1 receptor blockade results in decreased blood pressure, decreased resting heart rate, vasodilatation and decrease in peripheral resistance (causing orthostatic hypotension).
   b ECG changes like ↑ QT-PT interval; flattening or notching of P wave; ST segment depression; ventricular tachycardia (VT) – caused by local anaesthetic effect; quinidine-like effects.
3 *Miscellaneous effects*: Local anaesthetic effect; hypothermia; renal effects (e.g. ↓ADH secretion → ↓ Na⁺ and Cl⁻ absorption); hepatic effects (e.g. cholestatic jaundice because of swelling of canaliculi); antihistaminic like effects (e.g. sedation); skeletal muscle relaxant effect (no effect is produced on the neuromuscular junction).

Lithium carbonate

Effects on electrolytes and ion transport: Lithium is closely related to Na⁺ in its properties. It can substitute for Na⁺ in generating action potentials and in Na⁺-Na⁺ exchange across the membrane. It inhibits the latter process, i.e. Li-Na⁺ exchange is gradually slowed after lithium is introduced into the body. At therapeutic concentrations (around 1mmol/L), it does not significantly effect the Na⁺/Ca⁺⁺ exchange process or Na⁺/K⁺ ATPase pump.

    Effects on neurotransmitters: Lithium appears to enhance some of the actions of serotonin though findings have been contradictory. Its effects on norepinephrine are variable. The drug may decrease norepinephrine and dopamine turnover and these effects, if confirmed, might be relevant to its antimanic actions. Lithium also appears to block the development of dopamine receptor supersensitivity that may accompany chronic therapy with antipsychotic agents. Finally lithium may augment the synthesis of acetylcholine perhaps by increasing choline uptake into nerve terminals.

Effects on second messengers: One of the best defined effects of lithium is its action on inositol phosphates. Inositol-1, 4, 5-triphosphate (IP_3) and diacylglycerol (DAG) are important second messengers for both α-adrenergic and muscarinic transmission. Lithium inhibits several important enzymes in the normal recycling of the membrane phosphoinositides including the conversion of IP_2 to IP_1 (inositolmonophosphate) and the conversion of IP_1 to inositol. This block leads to the depletion of phosphatidylinositol-4,5-biphosphate (PIP_2), which is the membrane precursor of IP_3 and DAG. Over time the effects of transmitters on the cell diminish in proportion to the amount of activity in the PIP_2-dependent pathways. Before therapy, such activity might be greatly increased in mania. Thus lithium could cause a selective depression of the overactive circuits.

Effects on adenylyl cyclase: Studies of noradrenergic effects in isolated brain tissue indicate that lithium can inhibit norepinephrine sensitive adenylyl cyclase. Such an effect could relate to both its antidepressant and its antimanic effects.

Tricyclic antidepressants (TCAs)

These drugs block the reuptake of serotonin (5HT) and noradrenaline by blocking 5HT and α_2 presynaptic receptors respectively and by stimulating the presynaptic β_1 receptors present on the serotinergic and noradrenergic terminals. They do not affect the storage or synthesis of these amines. As a result of blockade of reuptake of these amines, their deficiency is made up in the brain relieving the symptoms of depression. Biochemical deficiency of these monoamines is made up within 24–48hrs during the treatment; however, therapeutic effects appear after 2–3 weeks. During this lag period, adaptive changes in the adrenergic, serotinergic and histaminic receptors takes place, which include:

Presynaptic receptor adaptive changes:

A Presynaptic α_2 and $5HT_1$ receptors are downregulated increasing the release of noradrenaline and 5HT respectively by knocking out negative feedback on the release of these hormones.

B Presynaptic β_1 receptors are upregulated increasing positive feed back on release of noradrenaline.

Postsynaptic receptor adaptive changes:

A β_1, β_2 and $5HT_2$ receptors are downregulated while H_2 receptors are either blocked or downregulated in the CNS.

B α_1 receptors in the CNS may be upregulated or no change occurs in them. However, α_1 receptors in blood vessels may be blocked leading to postural hypotension.

Precautions with the use of TCAs:

1 TCAs undergo variable first-pass metabolism in the liver with resultant inconsistent bioavailability. Because of this, their dose needs off-and-on adjustment.

2 TCAs have a narrow therapeutic index (a dose 5–6 times greater than the maximum daily dose of imipramine can be lethal). Therefore, depressed patients with suicidal tendency should not be given TCAs, or be given TCAs in low doses with vigilant monitoring.

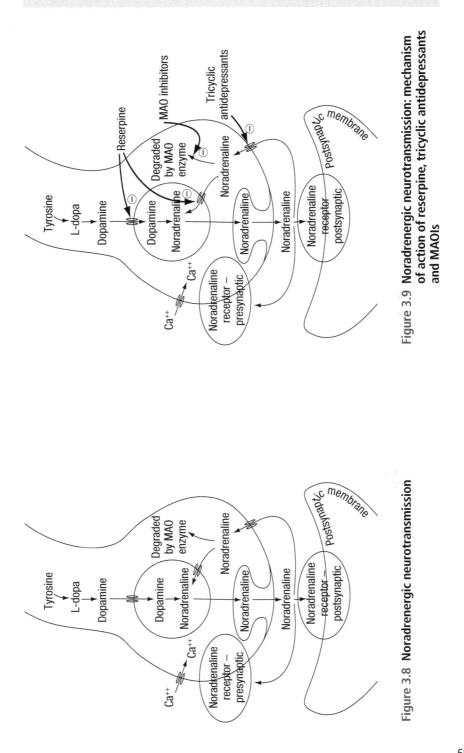

Figure 3.9 **Noradrenergic neurotransmission: mechanism of action of reserpine, tricyclic antidepressants and MAOIs**

Figure 3.8 **Noradrenergic neurotransmission**

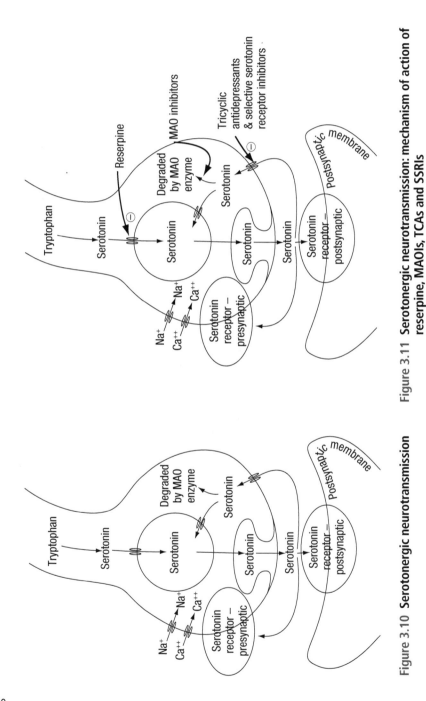

Figure 3.11 Serotonergic neurotransmission: mechanism of action of reserpine, MAOIs, TCAs and SSRIs

Figure 3.10 Serotonergic neurotransmission

3 Also, because they unmask the manic behaviour, they should be cautiously used in manic-depressive patients.

Selective serotonin re-uptake inhibitors (SSRIs)

As the name suggests these drugs block the pre-synaptic re-uptake of the serotonin with resultant greater post-synaptic neuronal activity. Unlike TCAs, which block the reuptake of both serotonin (5HT) and noradrenaline (by blocking 5HT and α_2 presynaptic receptors respectively), SSRIs have 300- to 3000-fold greater selectivity for 5HT receptors and thus primarily block the re-uptake of serotonin. Also, they have little ability to block the dopaminergic, muscarinic, α-adrenergic and histaminic (H_1) receptors. Because of this, SSRIs lack many of the side effects commonly encountered with TCA therapy, e.g. sedation, blurred vision, dry mouth and orthostatic hypotension. Fewer side effects, and being relatively safe even in high doses, have made SSRIs the drug of choice in most patients of depression in preference to TCAs and MAOIs.

SSRIs do not produce CNS stimulation or mood elevation in healthy subjects.

Monoamine oxidase inhibitors (MAOIs)

Monoamine oxidase (MAO) is a mitochondrial enzyme found in the neurons (and other tissues such as gut and liver). In the neurons, MAO functions as a safety valve to oxidatively deaminate and thus inactivate any excess neurotransmitter molecules (serotonin, noradrenaline and dopamine) that may leak out of the synaptic vesicles when the neuron is at rest. MAOIs may irreversibly or reversible inactivate both monoamine oxidase enzymes (MAO-A and MAO-B) by forming a strong covalent bond with the active sites of these enzymes. This results in inhibition of intraneuronal degradation of serotonin, noradrenaline and dopamine with resultant increase in the vesicular stores of these amines. When neuronal activity discharges the vesicles, increased amounts of the amines are released in the synaptic cleft causing enhanced activation of serotonin, noradrenaline and dopamine receptors. This may be responsible for the antidepressant actions of MAOIs. Notably, these MAOIs do not affect the synthesis and reuptake of the said amines.

MAOIs not only inhibit MAO in the brain, but also peripheral oxidases that catalyse oxidative deamination of drugs and potentially toxic substances such as tyramine, which is found in certain foods. MAOIs therefore show a high incidence of drug–drug and drug–food interactions.

Two MAOIs currently available for the treatment of depression are phenelzine and tranylcypromine. Besides inhibiting MAO, both these drugs show a direct (though mild), amphetamine-like stimulant effect. This makes theses drugs the preferred choice in depressed patients with low psychomotor activity. Also, they are indicated in depressed patients with associated severe anxiety, patients who are unresponsive or allergic to TCAs and patient's suffering from phobias or atypical depression.[3]

Levodopa

Since Parkinsonism results from dopamine deficiency in specific regions of the brain, attempts have been made to replenish the deficient dopamine.

---

3 Atypical depression is characterised by labile mood, appetite disturbances and rejection sensitivity.

Levodopa is rapidly absorbed from the small intestine (when empty of food), crosses BBB actively[4] and reaches nigrostriatal pathway[5]. It is taken up by substantia nigra and converted there into dopamine by cerebral dopa decarboxylase. Dopamine is released from N-terminal into striatal area thus making up dopamine deficiency and restoring the balance between dopamine and acetylcholine. This helps control the manifestations of Parkinsonism.

Large doses of levodopa are required because much of the drug is decarboxylated to dopamine in GIT and peripheral tissues resulting in side effects (like N, V, cardiac arrhythmias and hypotension). The effects of the levodopa on the CNS can be greatly enhanced by coadministering carbidopa (dopa decarboxylase inhibitor that does not cross the BBB). Carbidopa diminishes the metabolism of levodopa in the GIT and peripheral tissues hence increasing the CNS availability of levodopa. Addition of carbidopa lowers the doses of levodopa required by 4- to 5-folds and also decreases the severity of side effects of peripherally formed dopamine.

Levodopa has an extremely short half-life of 1–2hrs, which causes fluctuations in plasma concentration. This may produce fluctuations in motor response (on-off phenomenon), which may cause sudden worsening of the previously controlled Parkinsonian symptoms (loss of normal mobility, rigidity, tremors, and cramps).

Note that although levodopa meets dopamine deficiency in the brain, it does not stop the loss of dopaminergic neurons in the nigrostriatal pathway. This loss continues unchecked as the disease progresses so that after a given time very few dopaminergic neurons are left intact to take up levodopa for onward conversion to dopamine. Thus although levodopa produces a remarkable improvement in the symptoms during the initial period of therapy, its overall therapeutic efficacy declines with time.

Ingestion of meals particularly if high in protein content interferes with the transport of levodopa into the CNS. Large neutral amino acids, e.g. leucine and isoleucine compete with levodopa for absorption from the gut and for transport across the BBB. Thus levodopa should be taken on an empty stomach, typically 45 minutes before a meal.

Withdrawal from the drug must be gradual.

Penicillins

As antibacterial drugs, mechanism of action of all penicillins is the same. Penicillins are bactericidal and act by inhibiting the cell wall synthesis of the susceptible bacteria by blocking transpeptidation/cross links between the peptidoglycan chains through the inhibition of the enzymes transpeptidases. This renders the cell walls very weak resulting in loss of its protection to inner cytoplasmic membrane of the bacteria, which then bulges out under the high intracellular osmotic pressure and finally bursts out throwing its contents, i.e. essential macromolecules outside the cell. Thus death/lysis of bacterial cells occur.

Penicillins cause activation of autolysins by removing autolysin inhibitors. Autolysins on becoming active start destroying the bacterial cell wall. In order to inhibit transpeptidases, penicillins have to reach their targets, i.e. penicillins binding proteins (PBP) located on inner cytoplasmic membranes. They enter through the hydrophilic poring

---

4 Dopamine itself does not cross the BBB.

5 Nigrostriatal pathway is the extrapyramidal center where most dopaminergic neurons are concentrated. In Parkinsonism, dopaminergic neurons are partly lost, resulting in atrophy of the nigrostriatal pathway.

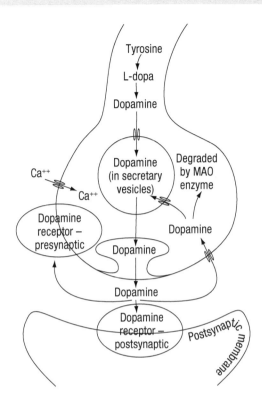

Figure 3.12 **Dopaminergic neurotransmission**

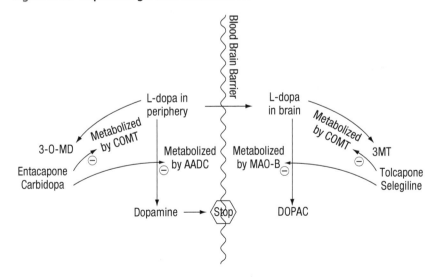

Figure 3.13 **Mechanism of action of levodopa and other anti-Parkinsonism drugs**

channels in outer membrane of bacteria. It is believed that beta-lactam ring (6-amino-penicillanic acid nucleus) of the bacteria is a structural analogue of D-alanyl-D-alanine. During transpeptidation in the presence of penicillins, beta-lactam ring is incorporated in the cross links rather than D-alanyl-D-alanine and this renders that cross links between peptidoglycan chains weak.

Cephalosporins

1 They bind to specific penicillin biding protein (PBP)-receptors on bacteria causing inhibition of cell wall synthesis by blocking transpeptidation of peptidoglycans.
2 They also cause activation of autolytic enzymes in the cell wall causing bacterial death.

Sulfonamides

They are bacteriostatic and inhibit protein synthesis. Sulfonamide susceptible organisms, unlike mammals, cannot use exogenous folate but must synthesise it from PABA.

This pathway is essential for the synthesis of purines and nucleic acids. Since sulfonamides are structural analogues of PABA, they inhibit dihydropteroate synthase and thus folate production. Sulfonamides inhibit both gram positive and negative bacteria. Rickettsiae are not inhibited, rather stimulated by sulfonamides. Combination of a sulfonamide with an inhibitor of dihydrofolate reductase (like trimethoprim) provides synergistic activity because of sequential inhibition of folate synthesis.

Tetracyclines

Tetracyclines are bacteriostatic and act by inhibiting bacterial protein synthesis at ribosomal level. They reach their site of action (30S ribosomal subunit of susceptible bacteria) through cell membrane 'porin' channels by simple diffusion or by active energy-dependent transport process. They bind reversibly to 30S ribosomal subunit and block biding of amino-acyl tRNA to the receptor site on mRNA-ribosomal complex. Addition of amino acids to the growing peptide chain is prevented thus inhibiting protein synthesis producing bacteriostatic effect.

Tetracyclines also interfere with oxidative phosphorylation, glucose oxidation, bacteria respiration and cell permeability.

Quinolones

They are bactericidal and block bacterial DNA synthesis by inhibiting the following enzymes:
1 DNA gyrase (topoisomerase-II).
2 Topoisomerase-IV.

Chloramphenicol

It is *bacteriostatic* for all susceptible microorganisms by protein synthesis inhibition at ribosomal level by binding reversibly to 50S ribosomal subunit near the binding site for macrolides and clindamycin (thus these drugs can interfere with each others actions). Chloramphenicol inhibits binding of amino acids containing aminoacyl tRNA to the acceptor site of the mRNA-ribosomal complex. Interaction between peptidyl transferase and its amino acid substrate is prevented. Amino acids are not added to the growing peptide chain so protein synthesis is inhibited.

Chloramphenicol may be *bactericidal* for *Haemophilus influenzae, Nisseria meningitidis* and some strains of bacteroides.

Amoebicides

Amoebicides irreversibly inhibit protein synthesis by blocking the movement of ribosomes along mRNA. They act only against amoebic trophozoites.

Aminoglycosides

They are bactericidal against aerobic, Gram –ve bacteria and some Gram +ve cocci. Aminoglycosides are irreversible inhibitors of protein synthesis. The initial event is passive diffusion via poring channels across the out membrane. Drug is then actively transported across the inner membrane into the cytoplasm by an oxygen-dependent process. The transmembrane electrochemical gradient supplies the energy for this process and transport is coupled to a proton pump. Low extracellular pH and anaerobic conditions inhibit the transport by reducing the gradient. Transport may be enhanced by drugs which inhibit cell wall synthesis such as β-lactam penicillins or vancomycin. This enhancement may be the basis of synergism of these antibiotics with aminoglycosides. Once inside the cytoplasm, aminoglycosides bind to specific 30S ribosomal subunit proteins (S12 in case of streptomycin). Protein synthesis is inhibited in at least three ways:

1 Aminoglycosides distort the structure of 30S ribosomal subunit, thus interfering with the initiation of protein synthesis.
2 Misreading of mRNA, which causes incorporation of incorrect amino acids into the peptide resulting in the formation of nonfunctional or toxic proteins.
3 Break up of polysomes into nonfunctional monosomes.

These activities occur more or less simultaneously and the overall effect is irreversible and lethal for the cell.

Aminoglycosides also damage inner cytoplasmic membrane by incorporating defective proteins in the cytoplasmic bacterial membrane. The membrane loses its permeability throwing small and large molecules (structural and functional proteins) leading to bacterial cell death. This is called energy-dependent phase-II transport.

Macrolides

At usual doses, macrolides are bacteriostatic; at higher doses, however, they become bactericidal. Their binding site is either the same or in close proximity to that of clindamycin and chloramphenicol. These drugs bind with 50S subunit of the bacterial ribosome thus inhibiting the translocation step of protein synthesis. Additionally, they may also interfere with the transpeptidation step.

Metronidazole

This drug is particularly effective against anaerobic protozoan parasites (including entamoeba histolytica, etc.). These organisms possess electron-transport proteins that participate in electron removal reactions. The nitro group of metronidazole acts as an 'electron acceptor' resulting in formation of cytotoxic compounds that bind to proteins and DNA rendering them nonfunctional. This leads to cell death.

Clonidine

Clonidine, being lipid soluble, crosses the BBB by simple diffusion and is taken up by the adrenergic neurons and the vasomotor centre of the brain. It is an active drug unlike α-methyl dopa, which is a pro-drug. Clonidine acts as an agonist on α_2-receptors situated post-synaptically on the neurons. These α-receptors are α_{2A} in nature. When stimulated, they cause increase in the negative feedback on the release of noradrenaline in brain stem resulting in decreased release from centre to periphery mainly in the heart. This causes fall in blood pressure especially in supine and upright positions by causing decrease in the force of contraction and heart rate leading to decrease in cardiac output. Bradycardia is more marked due to stimulation of parasympathetic system by the drug. Fall in blood pressure is accompanied by decrease in the concentration of noradrenaline and renin in the plasma. Postural hypotension is very mild and is seen in hypovolemic patients only. This is because of agonist effect on the peripheral α_{2B} and α_1 adrenergic receptors. In smooth muscles of blood vessels, it acts as an agonist causing vasoconstriction.

Alpha-methyl dopa

It is a structural analogue of levodopa. It is usually given orally. Its absorption through GIT is incomplete. The drug crosses the BBB by an active transport process responsible for the transport of aromatic amino acids. After having reached the brain, it is taken up by adrenergic neurons in the brain stem area where it is converted into α-methyl nor-dopamine, which in turn is converted into α-methyl nor-epinephrine. This process of conversion goes on side by side both in brain and in peripheral sympathetic adrenergic neurons. So it is concentrated in the intraneuronal granules in brain and in periphery and is stored there displacing noradrenaline from the storage vesicles. It is released as α-methyl epinephrine both in centre and in periphery. In periphery, it acts as α_1 post-synaptic receptor agonist leading to vasoconstriction and increase in blood pressure. It does not act as antihypertensive peripherally. In the brain, α-methyl nor-epinephrine acts as agonist at α_2 post-synaptic receptors causing increase in the negative feedback on release of noradrenaline. So less noradrenaline is released resulting in decreased sympathetic flow from centre to periphery. Methyl dopa mainly produces its antihypertensive effects by causing vasodilatation and decreasing total peripheral resistance by causing variably reduction in heart rate and blood pressure.

$\beta2$ selective adrenoceptor agonist drugs

These drugs are given by inhalational, oral and parenteral routes. They are β_2 selective adrenoceptor agonists and cause bronchodilatation.

Methylxanthines

In high concentrations in vitro, they inhibit several members of phosphodiesterase (PDE) enzyme family. Since phosphodiesterases hydrolyse cyclic nucleotides, this inhibition results in higher concentration of intracellular cAMP and in some tissues cGMP. cAMP is responsible for a myriad of cellular functions including:

1 Stimulation of cardiac functions.
2 Relaxation of smooth muscles.
3 Reduction in the immune and inflammatory activity of specific cells.

In the PDE enzyme family, amongst the various isoforms of phosphodiesterases,

PDE4 appears to be the most directly involved in the actions of methylxanthines on airway smooth muscle and on inflammatory cells. The inhibition of PDE4 in inflammatory cells reduces their release of cytokines and chemokines, which in turn results in a decrease in immune cell migration and activation.

Another proposed mechanism is inhibition of cell surface receptors for adenosine. These receptors modulate adenylyl cyclase activity, and adenosine has been shown to provoke contraction of isolated airway smooth muscle and histamine release from airway mast cells.

Corticosteroids (as antiasthmatics)

At biochemical level: Corticosteroids decrease the production of pro-inflammatory mediators (like cytokines, leukotrienes, prostaglandins, platelet-activating factor, etc.).

At cellular level: Corticosteroids inhibit the proliferation of T-lymphocytes and are cytotoxic to certain subsets of T-cells ($\rightarrow \downarrow$ cellular immunity). They also increase the catabolism of IgG ($\rightarrow \downarrow$ humoral immunity).

In asthmatics, corticosteroids do not directly cause bronchodilatation. In fact, by decreasing the production and release of pro-inflammatory mediators they reduce bronchial reactivity to different allergens and thus cause a reduction in the frequency of asthma exacerbations.

Besides decreasing the production and release of pro-inflammatory mediators, corticosteroids also cause contraction of engorged vessels in the bronchial mucosa. They also potentiate the effects of β- agonists on the airways.

Mast cell stabilisers

Mast cell stabilisers cause alteration in the function of delayed Cl⁻ channels in the cell membrane inhibiting cell activation. This action on airway nerves is thought to be responsible for nedocromil's inhibition of cough on:

A Mast cells for inhibition of early response to antigen challenge.

B Eosinophils for inhibition of inflammatory response to inhalation of allergens.

The inhibitory effect on mast cells appears to be specific for cell type since cromolyn has little inhibitory effect on mediator release from human basophils. It may also be specific for different organs, since cromolyn inhibits mast cells degranulation in human and primate lungs but in the skin. This in turn may reflect known differences in mast cells found at different sites as in their neutral protease content.

Leukotriene pathway inhibitors

They either cause inhibition of 5-lipoxygenase thereby preventing leukotriene synthesis or cause inhibition of binding of LTD$_4$ to its receptor on target tissues, thereby preventing its action.

Adrenocorticosteroids

They enter the cell and bind to cytosolic receptors that transport the steroid into the nucleus. The steroid-receptor complex alters gene expression by binding to glucocorticoid response elements (GREs) or mineralocorticoid-specific elements. Tissue specific responses to steroids are made possible by the presence in each tissue of different protein regulators that control the interaction between the hormone receptor complex and particular response element.

Heparin

Heparin is a heterogeneous mixture of sulfated mucopolysaccharides. It binds to antithrombin-III (ATIII) forming a heparin-ATIII complex. This complex binds and irreversibly inactivates thrombin (activated factor II), factors IXa, Xa, XIa, XIIa, and XIIIa. In the presence of heparin, ATIII proteolyses clotting factors 1000-fold faster than in its absence.

Warfarin

Warfarin inhibits Vit-K dependent synthesis of factors X, VII, IX and X in the liver by inhibiting the enzyme Vit-K epoxide reductase.

Hormonal contraception (oral/parenteral/implanted)

Combination pills: The combinations of oestrogens and progestins exert their contraceptive effect largely through selective inhibition of pituitary functions that results in inhibition of ovulation. They also produce a change in the cervical mucus, uterine endometrium, motility and secretion in fallopian tubes. All these changes decrease the likelihood of conception and implantation.

Progestins alone pills: Continuous use of progestins alone does not always inhibit ovulation. The other factors mentioned therefore play a major role in the prevention of pregnancy when these agents are used.

Postcoital pills: The exact mechanism of action is not well understood. However, it appears that they inhibit LH surge thus inhibiting ovulation. They probably also produce the same changes in the cervical mucus, uterine endometrium and fallopian tubes as being produced by the combination pills.

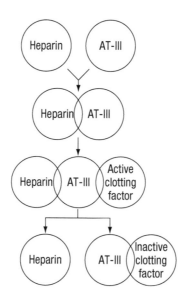

Figure 3.14 **Mechanism of action of heparin and antithrombin-III (AT-III)**

Organic nitrates and nitrites

1 *Biochemical*: When these drugs are taken orally, they are denitrated in the body (especially in the vascular and liver bed of endothelium) in a stepwise fashion. Initially one radical is removed, then another, by glutathione iso-reductase enzyme. Hydrolysis takes place and metabolites are released.

Release of nitric oxide radical → activation of guanylyl (guanylate) cyclase → accumulation of cGMP → activation of cGMP dependent kinases → dephosphorylation of myosin light chain → vasodilatation (venular and arteriolar).

2 *Hemodynamic*: venodilatation → decreased preload → arteriolar dilatation → decreased.

Phosphodiesterase (PDE) inhibitors

Phosphodiesterase (PDE) inhibitors (Sildena*fil*, tadala*fil*, vardena*fil*) fill the penis with blood and are thus used in men with erectile dysfunction. Physiologically, NO released from penile nerve terminals stimulates guanylyl cyclase in the smooth muscle of corpus cavernosum → ↑ intracellular cGMP → smooth muscle relaxation → ↑ inflow of blood → erection. It is pertinent to mention here that if we artificially increase the in vivo NO level by coadministering nitrates and PDE inhibitors, generalised vasodilatation and profound hypotension may result. Thus prescribing PDE inhibitors in patients who are taking nitrates (say due to unstable angina) is contraindicated.

Radioactive iodine I^{131} therapy

I^{131} is administered orally in solution form as sodium I^{131}. It is absorbed rapidly, after which it is avidly taken up by the thyroid tissue and incorporated in the storage follicles. I^{131} destroys thyroidal tissue by the emission of β-rays, which are cytotoxic, ionising and have got short-range (so destroy only follicle cells, not surrounding structures). They have an effective t½ of 5 days and a penetration range of 400–2000µm.

Unlike thioamides and iodine salts, which decrease thyroid hormone synthesis and/or release only transiently, I^{131} causes complete destruction of thyroid tissue within a few weeks producing permanent hypothyroidism and a cure to thyrotoxicosis without surgery.

Being radioactive, I^{131} therapy is contraindicated in pregnant ladies and lactating mothers.

Indications of I^{131} therapy

Thyrotoxicosis due to:
1 Graves' disease.
2 Toxic multi-nodular goitre.
3 Toxic nodule.

I^{131} is the only isotope used for the treatment of thyrotoxicosis; others are used in diagnosis. It is the drug of choice for the treatment of Graves' disease in patients <35yrs of age (except in pregnant/lactating women, in whom it is contraindicated).

Advantages of I^{131} therapy

1 Because of once daily dosage, I^{131} has good compliance.
2 Being odourless, it is not unpleasant to take it.

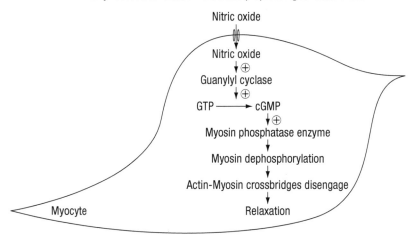

Figure 3.15 Mechanism of vascular smooth muscle relaxation

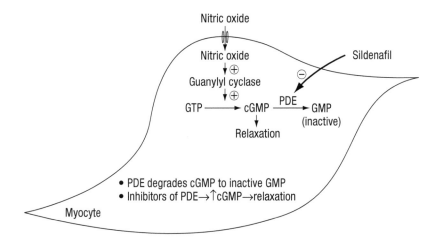

Figure 3.16 Mechanism of action of phosphodiesterase (PDE) inhibitors

3 It is cost-effective.

4 It is safe (mortality is rare). Fears of radiation-induced genetic damage, leukaemia or neoplasia have not been realised after >50yrs of clinical experience with radio-iodine therapy.

5 It is a painless procedure, done in an OPD. No hospitalisation of patient is required and thus no work loss is incurred.

6 Patient is saved from the hazards of surgery.

Thyroid hormone synthesis and transport

Synthesis of both triiodothyronine (T_3) and thyroxine (T_4) requires iodine, which is derived from food and iodine supplements (iodine-fortified salt, etc.). Iodine is taken up by the thyroid gland by an active process. Once inside the thyroid gland, the iodide ion combines with tyrosine to form monoiodotyrosine (MIT) and diiodotyrosine (DIT). Next, two molecules of DIT combine to form T_4, and one molecule each of MIT and DIT combine to form T_3. Once synthesised, these hormones are stored in the thyroid gland. On their release, both T4 and T3 circulate in the blood combined with a protein called thyroxine-binding globulin (synthesised by the liver). In peripheral tissues, some of the T_4 is converted to T_3 by a process of deiodination. Although T_3 is released as such by the thyroid gland also, most of the circulating T_3 comes by this process of deiodination of T_4 to T_3. T_3 is about 10 times more potent than T_4. It is basically T_3 that exerts most of the physiological effects of thyroid hormones at the target organs.

Thyroid-stimulating hormone (TSH) released by the pituitary gland stimulates T_4 and T_3 synthesis by the thyroid gland. Higher levels of T_4 and T_3 in turn inhibit pituitary release of TSH thus providing an effective negative feedback control mechanism.

Antithyroid drugs: thioamides

Drugs included: propylthiouracil; carbimazole.

These drugs inhibit the synthesis (not release) of thyroid hormones. They block the process of T_4 and T_3 synthesis at multiple points:

1 They inhibit iodination of the tyrosine residues.

2 They block the coupling of MIT and DIT.

3 Propylthiouracil alone, when given in high doses, also blocks the peripheral conversion of T_4 to T_3.

Since these drugs only inhibit the synthesis of thyroid hormones (and not release), their pharmacological effects starts only when the already synthesised and stored thyroid hormone molecules are depleted. This takes about 3–4 weeks.

Iodide salts and iodine

These drugs decrease both the synthesis (by inhibiting the iodination of tyrosine) and release of thyroid hormones. Because of the latter effect, unlike thioamides, these drugs have a rapid onset of action (within 2–7 days). Additionally, these drugs also decrease the size and vascularity of the enlarged hyperplastic thyroid gland. They are thus most beneficial when given in the pre-op period when, by decreasing the vascularity of the thyroid gland, they decrease the chances of per-op and post-op haemorrhage from the thyroid tissue.

The effects of iodide salts and iodine are transient. After a few weeks, the thyroid gland stops responding and escapes from the iodide block rendering these drugs ineffective.

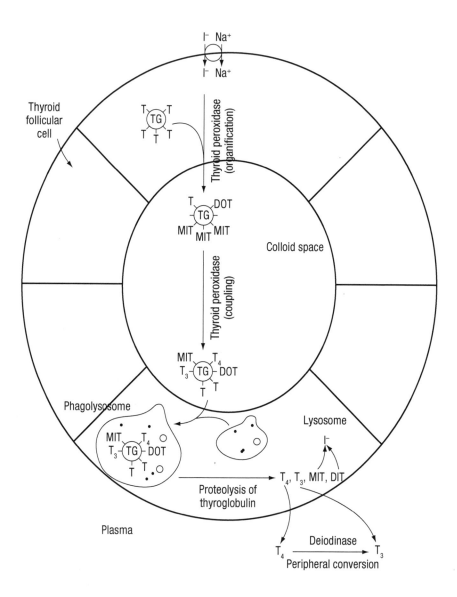

Figure 3.17 **Thyroid hormones synthesis, storage and release**

These drugs are usually given in the form of Lugol's solution (iodine and potassium iodide).

Aspirin and NSAIDs

As we know that arachidonic acid (derived from the cell membrane lipids) metabolism follows two pathways – lipoxygenase and cyclooxygenase. The latter pathway leads to the formation of three eicosanoids, i.e. prostacyclin, prostaglandins (PGE and PGF) and thromboxane.

Cyclooxygenase (COX) enzyme exists in 2 isoforms – COX-1 and COX-2. COX-1 is found in many body tissues, primarily in the non-inflammatory cells; COX-2, however, is found primarily in the inflammatory cells (polymorphonuclear cells, lymphocytes, etc.).

Aspirin and other non-selective NSAIDs: inhibit both COX-1 and COX-2 in turn inhibiting the synthesis of eicosanoids throughout the body. Eicosanoids are important mediators of inflammation. For example, they are involved in increasing or decreasing vascular and bronchial tone, leukocyte chemotaxis, platelet aggregation, etc. By inhibiting eicosanoids synthesis, these drugs exert their anti-inflammatory effect. For example, PG synthesis in CNS (stimulated by pyrogens) leads to fever. NSAIDs by suppressing PG synthesis, thus produce an antipyretic effect. PGs produced in the injured tissues activate the nociceptors. NSAIDs exert an analgesic effect by suppressing PG synthesis in the injured tissues. PG synthesis in the stomach protects the gastric lining from the cytotoxic effects of HCl. This cytoprotection is lost when PG synthesis is inhibited by the NSAIDs leading to gastritis and peptic ulceration.

Difference between aspirin and other non-selective NSAIDs: Unlike other non-selective NSAIDs, aspirin (but not its active metabolite, salicylate) acetylates and thus irreversibly inhibits COX-1 and COX-2 enzymes. This leads to a longer duration of action (especially the antiplatelet effect).

COX-2 selective NSAIDs (celecoxib and rofecoxib): only inhibit the COX-2 enzyme primarily found in the inflammatory cells. These agents thus do not inhibit eicosanoids synthesis throughout the body. Thus, at least theoretically, these agents should have lesser GI side effects (gastritis and peptic ulceration) – something not uncommonly seen with protracted therapy with aspirin and other non-selective NSAIDs.

GPIIb-IIIa receptor antagonists

Fibrinogen strands bind with GPIIb-IIIa receptors present on platelet membranes leading to platelet aggregation. GPIIb-IIIa receptor antagonists (like tirofiban and abciximab) by inhibiting GPIIb-IIIa receptors inhibit platelet aggregation. Use of these potent antiplatelet drugs is reserved in selected cases of unstable angina and non-ST elevation myocardial infarction (NTEMI) and those undergoing percutaneous coronary intervention.

Clopidogrel, ticlopidine and dipyridamole

cAMP is one of the *'natural antiplatelets'* found in human bodies. An *increase* in the intracellular concentration of cAMP in platelets leads to *decrease* platelet aggregation and vice versa (the exact mechanism not clearly understood). Physiologically, ADP receptor activation causes *inactivation* of adenylyl cyclase enzyme leading to a fall in cAMP levels. Drugs like clopidogrel and ticlopidine irreversibly inhibit the ADP

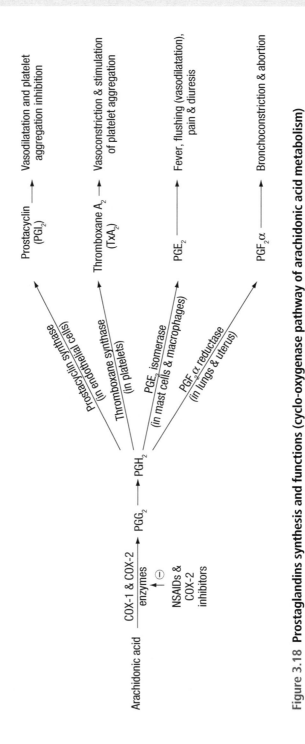

Figure 3.18 Prostaglandins synthesis and functions (cyclo-oxygenase pathway of arachidonic acid metabolism)

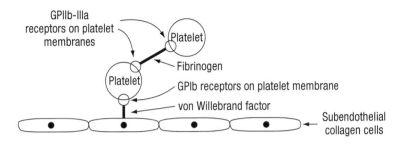

Platelets bind to vascular subendothelial collagen cells via von Willebrand factor. Platelets bind with each other via fibrinogen strands

Figure 3.19 Mechanism of platelets adhesion and aggregation

receptors present on platelet cell membranes in turn causing *activation* of adenylyl cyclase → ↑ intracellular cAMP → platelet aggregation inhibition. cAMP is degraded by phosphodiesterase (PDE) enzyme into inactive AMP. Dipyridamole, another antiplatelet drug, inhibits PDE → ↑ intracellular cAMP → platelet aggregation inhibition.

Methotrexate

As a DMARD: It is a disease-modifying antirheumatic drug (DMARD). It acts by inhibiting lymphoid proliferation and thus reducing the number of immune cells available to participate in the inflammatory response.

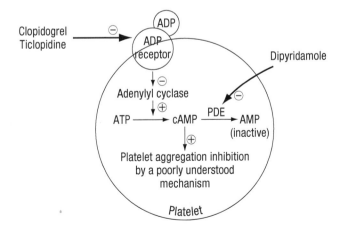

Figure 3.20 ADP-dependent pathway of platelet activation

As an anticancer drug: DNA synthetic pathway:
Methotrexate is a substrate for and inhibitor of dihydrofolate reductase. Inhibition of this enzyme blocks DNA synthesis at two points:
 1 It decreases the synthesis of purine and pyrimidine nucleotides.
 2 It decreases the synthesis of DNA from deoxynucleotides.

Cyclophosphamide
It is a prodrug that is transformed by hepatic cytochrome P450 enzymes to an alkylating agent. Just like other alkylating agents, cyclophosphamide is a cell cycle-nonspecific (CCNS) drug. It damages DNA by alkylating nucleophilic groups on DNA bases (particularly the N-7 position of guanine). This leads to cross-linking of bases, abnormal base pairing and ultimate breakage of DNA strands. Cyclophosphamide is cytotoxic to proliferating lymphoid cells – both B and T lymphocytes ($\rightarrow$ immunosuppression), although, effect on the former cells is greater.

Vincristine and vinblastine
Vinca alkaloids (vincristine and vinblastine) are cell cycle-specific agents that primarily act in the M phase of cancer cell cycle. They prevent the assembly of tubulin dimmers into microtubules. This in turn blocks the formation of mitotic spindles.

Doxorubicin and daunorubicin
These anthracyclines are cell cycle-nonspecific (CCNS) drugs. They intercalate between base pairs, inhibit topoisomerase II and generate free radicals. Free radicals in turn block the synthesis of RNA and DNA and cause scission of DNA strands.

Amphotericin B
It is a polyene antifungal agent. Polyene molecules are amphipathic, i.e. they are both hydrophilic and lipophilic. They bind to ergosterol (a sterol specifically found in the cell membranes of fungi) in turn causing the formation of artificial pores in fungal cell membranes. These pores allow leakage of intracellular ions and macromolecules eventually leading to cell death.

Nystatin
Just like amphotericin B, Nystatin is a polyene antifungal agent. Its mechanism of action is similar to that of amphotericin B.

Griseofulvin
It is taken up by sensitive dermatophytes by an energy-dependent mechanism. Once inside the cytoplasm, Griseofulvin interferes with microtubular function and inhibits synthesis and polymerisation of nucleic acids. The net result is death of dermatophytes.

Acyclovir
Acyclovir is a guanosine analogue. It is activated by a viral enzyme called thymidine kinase to form acyclovir triphosphate. The latter is incorporated into viral DNA, where it causes chain termination by inhibiting viral DNA polymerase.
 Since phosphorylation of acyclovir is necessary for its antiviral effect, viral strains

that lack thymidine kinase are resistant to acyclovir. Also, a change in viral DNA polymerase so that it is no longer inhibited by acyclovir triphosphate can cause viral resistance to acyclovir.

Metoclopramide

In the enteric nervous system (ENS), metoclopramide increases upper GI motility by:

1 Acting as an acetylcholine facilitator.

2 Acting as dopamine receptor antagonists.

The net effect is an increase in upper GI motility with resultant alleviation of vomiting.

Antiarrhythmic drugs

Table 3.3

Class	Example	Mnemonic: MBA college	Mechanism
Ia	Disopyramide	Membrane stabilisers (Na$^+$ channel blockage → membrane stabilisation)	Na$^+$ channel blockers (prolong the AP; intermediate dissociation)
Ib	Lidocaine	Membrane stabilisers (Na$^+$ channel blockage → membrane stabilisation)	Na$^+$ channel blockers (shorten the AP; fast dissociation)
Ic	Flecainide	Membrane stabilisers (Na$^+$ channel blockage → membrane stabilisation)	Na$^+$ channel blockers (no effect on AP duration; slow dissociation)
II	Propranolol	Beta blockers	β-Adrenoceptor blockers
III	Amiodarone, sotalol	Action potential widening agents (K$^+$ channel blockage → widening of AP)	K$^+$ channel blockers
IV	Verapamil	Calcium channel blockers	Ca^{++} channel blockers

Class	Example	PR interval	QRS duration	QT interval
Ia	Disopyramide	↓ or ↑*	↑↑	↑↑
Ib	Lidocaine	–	–	–
Ic	Flecainide	↑ (slightly)	↑↑	–
II	Propranolol	↑↑	–	–
III	Amiodarone, sotalol	↑ ↑	↑↑ –	↑↑↑↑ ↑↑↑
IV	Verapamil	↑↑	–	–
Misc	Adenosine	↑	–	–

*PR interval may ↓ d/t antimuscarinic action; it may ↑ d/t Na$^+$ channel blocking action

Calcium channel blockers

These drugs block voltage-gated 'L-type' Ca^{++} channels found in cardiac and other smooth muscle tissues $\rightarrow \downarrow Ca^{++}$ influx $\rightarrow \downarrow$ cytoplasmic Ca^{++} concentration $\rightarrow \downarrow$ muscle contractility (vasodilatation, and to a lesser extent dilatation of bronchial, gut and uterine smooth muscles). All Ca^{++} channels blockers reduce BP. Effect on heart rate is, however, variable. Diltiazem and verapamil block Ca^{++}-dependent AV nodal conduction $\rightarrow$ slowing of heart rate. Nifedipine and other dihydropyridines Ca^{++} channel blockers primarily affect the peripheral blood vessels $\rightarrow$ peripheral vasodilatation $\rightarrow \downarrow BP \rightarrow$ reflex tachycardia.

Note: Since 'L-type' Ca^{++} channels are not found at NM junctions and in endocrine tissues, Ca^{++} channel blockers do not affect the release of neurotransmitters or hormones.

K⁺ channel openers (minoxidil, nicorandil)

K^+ channel openers (minoxidil, nicorandil), as the name suggest, open K^+ channels present in the cell membranes of myocytes causing K^+ efflux. The resultant hyperpolarisation makes membrane depolarisation difficult to achieve by normal excitatory stimuli. In the absence of depolarisation, voltage gated Ca^{++} channels responsible for Ca^{++} influx do not open. The resultant fall in intracellular Ca^{++} leads to arterial smooth muscle relaxation.

Angiotensin-converting enzyme inhibitors (ACEIs)

Physiologic role of angiotensin-converting enzyme (ACE): ACE (also known as kininase-II and peptidyl dipeptidase) is responsible for the conversion of:

1 Angiotensin-I to angiotensin-II. The latter has three important effects:
   a It is a potent vasoconstrictor ($\rightarrow \uparrow$ peripheral vascular resistance).
   b It acts on angiotensin AT_1 receptors on the adrenal cortex and causes the release of aldosterone, which in turn causes Na^+ and water reabsorption in exchange of K^+ and H^+ from the distal convoluting tubules of the nephron.

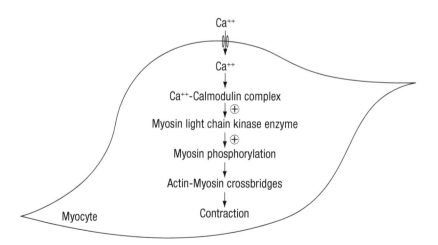

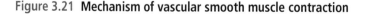

Figure 3.21 **Mechanism of vascular smooth muscle contraction**

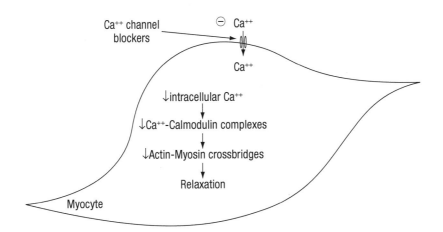

Figure 3.22 Mechanism of action of calcium channel blockers

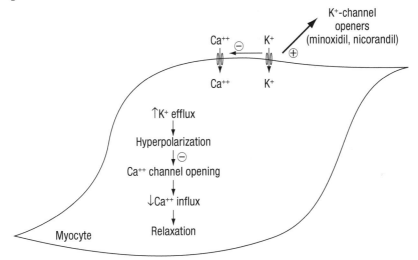

Figure 3.23 Mechanism of action of K+-channel openers (minoxidil, nicorandil)

    c It causes the release of norepinephrine from adrenergic nerve endings via presynaptic AT_1 receptor stimulation.

2 Bradykinin to inactive metabolites. Bradykinin is one of the most potent vasodilators known. It acts via at least two receptors – β_1 and β_2.

Effects of ACE Inhibition: ACE inhibition decreases the concentration of angiotensin-II (a vasoconstrictor and stimulant for aldosterone release) and increases the concentration of bradykinin (a vasodilator). The net effect is a fall in blood pressure (with minimal compensatory responses), and K^+ retention.

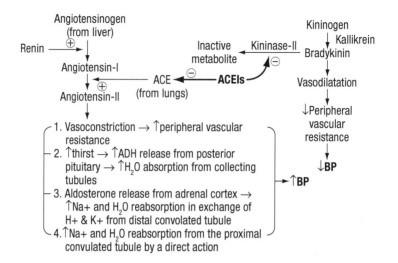

Figure 3.24 **Renin-angiotensin-aldosterone system**

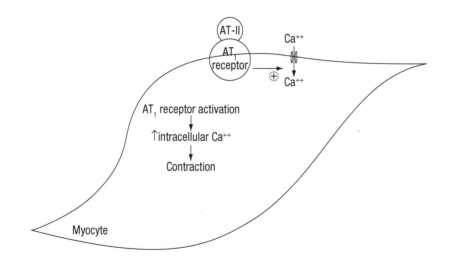

Figure 3.25 **Mechanism of angiotensin-II induced vasoconstriction**

Angiotensin receptor blockers (ARBs)

As the name suggests ARBs competitively inhibit angiotensin-II from acting at AT_1 receptors at adrenal cortex. They appear to be as effective as ACEIs in lowering the BP. Notably they do not block the conversion of bradykinin to inactive metabolites. Dry cough – a common side effect with ACEIs occurring in almost 30% cases – is due to a rise in the levels of bradykinin. Since ARBs lack this effect, they do not cause dry cough. In clinical practice, many patients who develop dry cough with ACEIs are switched to ARBs.

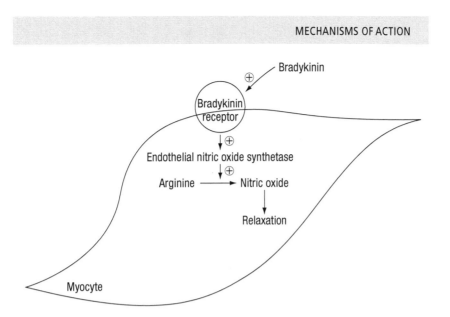

Figure 3.26 **Mechanism of bradykinin-induced vasodilatation**

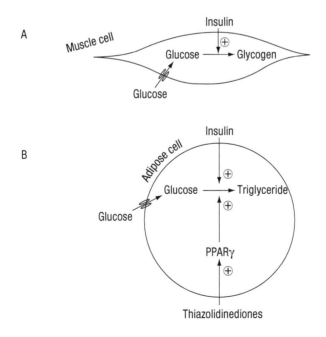

Figure 3.27 **A) Physiological action of insulin on muscle cells**
B) Physiological action of insulin on adipose cells

Since both ACEIs and ARBs cause K$^+$ retention, concomitant use of these drugs with K$^+$-sparing diuretics is not recommended lest toxic hyperkalemia should occur. Also, since both these groups of drugs damage the fetal kidneys, their use in pregnancy is absolutely contraindicated.

Sodium nitroprusside

Sodium nitroprusside is a short-acting (duration of action is a few minute), vasodilator always given as an intravenous infusion (never orally) in hypertensive emergencies. It produces its vasodilatory effect by causing the release of nitric oxide from the drug molecules itself, which in turn stimulates guanylyl cyclase and increases cGMP concentration in the smooth muscles.

Statins

Lovastatin and simvastatin are prodrugs; rest of the statins are active drugs. They inhibit hepatic synthesis of cholesterol by inhibiting an enzyme HMG-CoA reductase. 3-Hydroxy-3-methylglutaryl (HMG) is converted to mevalonate by an enzyme HMG-CoA reductase. This is the rate-limiting step in hepatic cholesterol biosynthesis. Statins by inhibiting HMG-CoA reductase in turn inhibit cholesterol biosynthesis leading to a fall in intracellular cholesterol concentration. Although cholesterol biosynthesis is blocked in other tissues as well, since statins undergo an extensive first-pass extraction, their primary effect is on liver. A fall in intracellular cholesterol concentration stimulates the synthesis of cell-surface LDL receptors. The resultant rise in the number of LDL receptors in turn causes an increased uptake of LDL cholesterol (the 'bad' cholesterol) from the blood. Statins thus reduce serum cholesterol levels by at least two mechanisms:

1 ↓ Hepatic cholesterol synthesis → ↓ hepatic cholesterol secretion into the blood.
2 ↑ LDL-cholesterol uptake from the blood.

The latter effect appears to be the more potent of the two in lowering serum cholesterol levels. Statins cause a rise in the level of HDL cholesterol (the 'good' cholesterol). The also decrease triglyceride levels.

Besides cholesterol-lowering effect, stains also have many other beneficial effects:
1 Atheromatous plaque-stabilising effect.[6]
2 Improvement in coronary endothelial function.
3 Prevention of platelet aggregation.
4 Anti-inflammatory effect.
5 Prevention of bone loss.

Fenofibrate

Fenofibrate is a prodrug. It is converted to an active metabolite 'fenofibric acid' which is responsible for the triglyceride-lowering effect of the drug. Fenofibric acid, once formed, attaches to its receptor: peroxisome proliferator-activated receptor-alpha

---

6 Atheromatous plaques usually only partly fill the vascular lumen. Complete luminal obstruction (with resultant infarction and tissue death) usually occurs when part of the atheromatous plaque is ruptured by the blood stream followed by clotting of blood on the raw surface of the ruptured plaque. By 'stabilising' the plaque, statins reduce the risk of plaque rupture.

(PPAR-α). The activated receptor then binds to peroxisome proliferator response elements located in various gene promoters. These elements increase the expression of genes encoding for lipoprotein lipase. This enzyme is primarily found on the surface of endothelial cells. Its main function is to clip off free fatty acids from within the lipoprotein complexes so that the same can be taken up into the cells. This leads to depletion of triglycerides (3 × fatty acids + glycerol) from the lipoprotein complexes. Increased expression of lipoprotein lipase means increased clearance of triglyceride-rich lipoproteins from the circulation leading to a fall in triglyceride levels. This also in turn leads to decreased cholesterol biosynthesis in the liver.

Fenofibrate also increases the level of HDL cholesterol (the 'good' cholesterol) by increasing the expression of two apolipoproteins apo A-I and apo A-II.

Insulin

Insulin synthesis: In the β-cells of the pancreas, insulin is initially synthesised as a prohormone called proinsulin (a single-chain polypeptide). It then undergoes proteolytic cleavage to form insulin (a two-chain polypeptide connected by disulfide bonds) and C-peptide, which are then secreted into the blood circulation. It is insulin that is responsible for all the physiological actions; neither proinsulin nor C-peptide appears to have any physiologic action.

Insulin secretion: A rise in blood glucose level, say after meals, causes increased glucose uptake by the β-cells of pancreas. Once inside the β-cells, glucose is metabolised. The products of glucose metabolism enter the mitochondrial respiratory chain generating ATP. A rise in ATP blocks K^+ channels leading to membrane depolarisation and an influx of Ca^{++}, which in turn causes insulin exocytosis. This explains a rise in insulin secretion following a rise in blood glucose level.

Box 3.2 Effects of insulin at target organs

Liver:	• ↑Glucose uptake • ↑Glycogen synthesis • ↓Glycogenolysis ↓Gluconeogenesis • ↓Protein catabolism
Muscles:	• ↑Glucose uptake • ↑Glycogen synthesis • ↓Glycogenolysis ↓Gluconeogenesis • ↑Protein synthesis (insulin builds up muscle mass)
Adipose tissue:	• ↑Glucose uptake • ↑Triglyceride storage • ↓Lipolysis (insulin builds up fat stores)

Net effect of the above-mentioned actions is a fall in the blood glucose level.

Chloroquine

Plasmodium fulfils its need for essential amino acids by digesting the host cells haemoglobin. This process occurs in the food vacuoles of the organism and releases large amounts of heme, which is ordinarily toxic to plasmodium. The organism

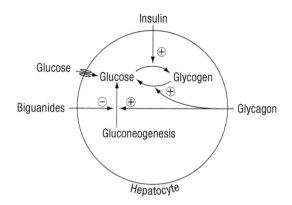

Figure 3.28 Effects of insulin, glucagon and biguanides on hepatocytes

protects itself from the toxic effects of heme by polymerising the heme to non-toxic hemozoin. Chloroquine is also concentrated in the food vacuoles where it binds to heme-polymerase preventing heme polymerisation. Heme accumulation results in oxidative damage to the membranes leading to lysis of the parasite.

It appears that quinidine and mefloquine also have the same mechanism of action.

Artemether

Artemether is a potent antimalarial drug used for the treatment of multi-drug resistant plasmodium falciparum infection and cerebral malaria. It is derived from Qinghaosu plant and has been in use in Chinese medicine since ancient times. Just like chloroquine, this drug preferentially concentrates in the food vacuoles of plasmodium, where it is metabolised to form toxic free radicals. Additionally, it appears that this drug covalently binds to specific malarial proteins, damaging and thus rendering them non-functional.

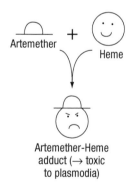

Figure 3.29 Mechanism of action of artemether

Digoxin

Digoxin, a cardiac glycoside, inhibits the Na^+/K^+ ATPase pump present in the cell membrane of cardiac myocytes. This pump normally causes Na^+ efflux in exchange of K^+ influx. A rise in ECF Na^+ in turn improves the gradient for Na^+ influx via the Na^+/Ca^{++} pump – another cell membrane pump responsible for Na^+ influx in exchange of Ca^{++} efflux. Digoxin, by inhibiting Na^+/K^+ ATPase pump, in turn decreases the activity of Na^+/Ca^{++} pump. The net effect is a rise in intracellular Ca^{++} so that when the digoxin-treated myocyte is depolarised, more Ca^{++} is available to facilitate contraction.

Besides the above-mentioned positive inotropic effect (increased *force* of contraction), digoxin also exerts a negative chronotropic effect (slowed *rate* of contraction) by a direct action on the cardiac conduction system. It prolongs the refractory period of AV node and slows the conduction velocity via the node.

Because of the characteristic electrophysiological effects of digoxin on heart, it is the drug of choice in treating atrial fibrillation (AF) in patients who have concomitant left ventricular failure. The aim of drug therapy in most AF patients is to slow the ventricular rate. Digoxin, by virtue of its negative chronotropic effect, achieves this aim, but unlike the other rate-controlling drugs used in AF (like β-blockers or rate-limiting Ca^{++} channel blockers like verapamil or diltiazem), it doesn't worsen the left ventricular failure (it *increases* the force of contraction, whereas other drugs *not only decrease the rate of contraction but also the force of contraction*).

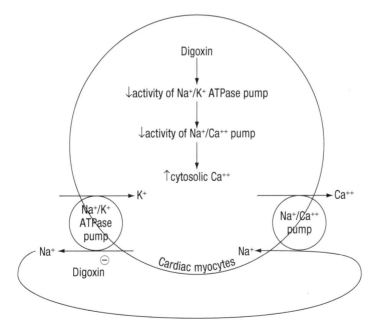

Figure 3.30 Mechanism of action of digoxin

95

4

Therapeutic uses and side effects

H-1 antagonists: therapeutic uses

1 *Allergic disorders*: Common cold, hayfever, seasonal rhinitis, conjunctivitis, urticaria, angioneurotic oedema, serum sickness, allergic drug reactions.
2 *Motion sickness* (cyclizine, meclizine).
3 *Ménière's disease and vertigo*.
4 *Vomiting* (promethazine and meclizine); chemotherapy-induced vomiting (diphenhydramine).

H-1 antagonists: side effects

1 *CNS*:
  - *Sedation* is common with the 1st generation antihistamines especially with diphenhydramine and promethazine. Pronounced sedation can occur if other drugs with sedative effect (like benzodiazepines, alcohol) are used concomitantly. Since 2nd generation antihistamines have poor CNS penetration, this side effect is much less common with the newer agents.
2 *Antimuscarinic effects*:
  - Like blurred vision, dryness of mouth/respiratory passages, constipation, urinary retention and orthostatic hypotension may occur, especially with some of the 1st generation antihistamines.
3 *Drug allergy*:
  - Acute poisoning is common in young children when they are given high doses. It is characterised by atropine-like antimuscarinic side effects.
4 *Blood dyscrasias*:
  - Leukopenia, agranulocytosis and haemolytic anaemia.

H-2 antagonists: therapeutic uses

1 *Peptic ulcer disease* (DU, GU, stress ulcers, NSAIDs-induced ulcers): They are also used both in the treatment and prophylaxis of bleeding peptic ulcers.
2 *GERD*.
3 *Syndromes*:
  a *Zollinger-Ellison syndrome* (hypergastrinemia → hypersecretion of gastric HCl → besides stomach and duodenum, peptic ulcers also develop at unusual sites like oesophagus and jejunum). Larger doses of H-2 antagonists are required; PPIs are more effective.

   b *Mendelson's syndrome* (acid aspiration syndrome).

   c *Short bowel anastomosis syndrome.*

DISCOS:
Digoxin
Isoniazid
Spironolactone
Cimetidine
Oestrogens
Stilboestrol

H-2 antagonists: side effects

1 *Anti-androgenic*: Cimetidine (alone) causes hyperprolactinemia. This in turn may lead to gynecomastia in males and galactorrhea in females.
2 *Hepatotoxicity*: As compared to ranitidine, cimetidine is a potent inhibitor of hepatic drug metabolising enzyme (CYP450). H-2 antagonists also reduce hepatic blood flow.
3 *Cardiotoxicity*: Bradycardia and hypotension.
4 *Blood dyscrasias*: Thrombocytopenia, granulocytopenia and hypoprothrombinemia.
5 *GIT*: Constipation, flatulence and diarrhoea.
6 *Miscellaneous*:
   a Opportunistic infections like candidal peritonitis.
   b Myalgias, arthralgias.

Proton Pump Inhibitors (PPIs): therapeutic uses

1 *Peptic ulcers* (DU, GU, stress ulcers, NSAIDs-induced ulcers): They are also used both in the treatment and prophylaxis of bleeding peptic ulcers.
2 *GERD.*
3 *Syndromes*:
   a Zollinger Ellison syndrome (hypergastrinemia → hypersecretion of gastric HCl → besides stomach and duodenum, peptic ulcers also develop at unusual sites like oesophagus and jejunum). PPIs (in high doses) are the most effective and thus preferred drugs in these cases.
   b Mendelson's syndrome (acid aspiration syndrome).
   c Short bowel anastomosis syndrome.
4 *H. pylori* (→ peptic ulcers, gastritis, gastric lymphoma) eradication.

Proton Pump Inhibitors: side effects

1 *GIT*:
   a NVD, flatulence and abdominal pain.
   b Hypergastrinemia (causing rebound hyper-secretion of gastric HCl) after discontinuation of PPI therapy.
   c Decreased absorption of vitamin B_{12} and certain drugs (e.g. digoxin, ketoconazole) that require acidity for their GI absorption.
   d Inhibition of hepatic CYP450 enzyme in turn causing decreased metabolism/clearance of BDZs, warfarin, phenytoin and many other drugs.
2 *Impotence.*
3 *Gynecomastia.*

4 *Subacute myopathy and arthralgias.*
5 *Skin rashes.*

Laxatives and purgatives: therapeutic uses
1 To relieve constipation.
2 In pathologies like haemorrhoids and anal fissures.
3 Expulsion of parasites after antihelminthic treatment.
4 To clear the gut before surgery/endoscopy/radiological examinations (like barium enema).
5 To induce labour, e.g. castor oil.

Bulk forming purgatives: therapeutic uses
1 Colostomy/ileostomy.
2 Constipation due to any cause like anal pathologies, e.g. haemorrhoids, anal fissures; IBD (ulcerative colitis); IBS (irritable bowel syndrome); diverticulitis.

Saline purgatives: therapeutic uses
1 Rapid bowel evacuation in 2–3hrs (6.5% solution).
2 I/V injection (CNS depressant).
3 Injection into the nerve ($\rightarrow$ blockade of impulse conduction).
4 10–20mL of 20% solution I/M abolishes convulsions.
5 Magnesium sulphate and glycerin paste (carbuncles).
6 50% retention enema (to decrease CSF in neurosurgery).

Bisacodyl: therapeutic uses
1 To relieve constipation.
2 To evacuate bowel pre-op, before endoscopy or any radiological procedure.

Castor oil: therapeutic uses
1 Emollient externally.
2 Soother for skin, conjunctiva and nasal mucosa.
3 Laxative. Since castor oil delays gastric emptying, it should be given on an empty stomach.

Thiazide diuretics: therapeutic uses
1 *Oedema* due to:
  a Cardiac cause (CCF).
  b Hepatic cause (cirrhosis).
  c Renal cause (CRF, nephrotic syndrome; acute glomerulonephritis).
2 *HTN* (primary, secondary, pre-eclampsia, i.e. pregnancy-induced hypertension).
3 *Hypercalciuria* ($\rightarrow$ recurrent renal stones formation): Thiazide diuretics decrease urinary calcium concentrations and thus are used to prevent renal stone formation.
4 *Halide poisoning* (bromide intoxication).

Mnemonic:
Thiazide diuretics: indications

'**CHIC** to use thiazides':
CHF
Hypertension
Insipidus
Calcium calculi

Thiazide diuretics: side effects

1 *Due to abnormalities of fluid and electrolyte balance*:
   a ECF volume depletion ($\rightarrow$ hypotension).
   b Hyponatremia.
   c Hypochloremia.
   d Hypokalemia.
   e Hypomagnesemia.
   f Hypophosphatemia.
   g Hypercalcemia (thiazide diuretics $\rightarrow$ all 'hypos' except hypercalcemia!).
   h Decreased plasma level of halides.
2 *Metabolic effects*:
   a Metabolic alkalosis.
   b Hyperglycemia.
   c Hyperuricemia.
   d Hyperlipidemia.
3 *Miscellaneous*:
   a CNS: Drowsiness.
   b GIT: NVD, constipation, acute pancreatitis and acute cholecystitis.
   c Allergic reactions: Photosensitivity and skin rashes.
   d Haematological reactions: Thrombocytopenia, neutropenia and haemolytic anaemia.
   e Sexual dysfunctions.

Loop diuretics: therapeutic uses

1 *Oedema* due to:
   a Cardiac cause (CCF)
   b Hepatic cause (cirrhosis)
   c Renal cause (CRF, nephrotic syndrome, AGN).
2 *HTN* (primary, secondary, pre-eclampsia, i.e. pregnancy-induced hypertension). Because of long duration of action, thiazide diuretics are the drugs of first choice in cases of HTN. If, however, response to thiazide diuretics is not adequate, loop diuretics can be used. *Note*: Short duration of action of loop diuretics is a disadvantage in this condition.
3 *Ascites* (collection of free fluid in the peritoneal cavity).
4 *Hypercalcemia* (e.g. secondary to malignancy). It is a potentially life-threatening condition. A combination of loop diuretics and intravenous fluids is required to correct this condition. Loop diuretics alone (without intravenous fluids) will cause haemoconcentration and may actually worsen hypercalcemia.
5 *Hyperkalemia*.
6 *Anion poisoning* (bromide, fluoride, iodide).

Loop diuretics: side effects

1 *Due to abnormalities of fluid and electrolyte balance*:
   a ECF volume depletion ($\rightarrow$ hypotension).
   b Hyponatremia.
   c Hypochloremia.
   d Hypokalemia.
   e Hypomagnesemia.
   f Hypophosphatemia.
   g Hypocalcemia (thiazide diuretics $\rightarrow$ hypercalcemia).
   h Decreased plasma level of halides.
2 *Metabolic effects*:
   a Metabolic alkalosis.
   b Hyperglycemia.
   c Hyperuricemia.
   d Hyperlipidemia.
3 *Miscellaneous*:
   a Ototoxicity: vertigo, dizziness, deafness, and changes in endolymph of ears.
   b Nephrotoxicity.
   c Hepatotoxicity.
   d Gynecomastia.
   e Allergic reactions (related to sulfonamide moiety): Photosensitivity, skin rashes and interstitial nephritis.

K⁺-sparing diuretics: therapeutic uses

1 Primary and secondary aldosteronism.
2 In order to prevent thiazide/loop diuretics-induced hypokalemia, K^+-sparing diuretics are used concomitantly. Thiazide/loop diuretics $\rightarrow \uparrow Na^+$ delivery to distal nephron $\rightarrow Na^+$ reabsorption in exchange of $K^+ \rightarrow$ hypokalemia; K^+-sparing diuretics block this Na^+/K^+ exchange $\rightarrow K^+$ retention.
3 Long-term treatment for refractory oedema as in cirrhosis.

Osmotic diuretics: therapeutic uses

1 As the name suggests they are used as diuretics ($\rightarrow$ water excretion $> Na^+$ excretion).
2 Muscular injury such as in RTA $\rightarrow$ rhabdomyolysis $\rightarrow$ myoglobulinuria $\rightarrow$ acute renal failure. Osmotic diuretics by facilitating myoglobulin excretion help prevent ARF.
3 Reduction of ICP and IOP.

Heparin: therapeutic uses

Because of its rapid onset of action, heparin is useful when an immediate anticoagulant effect is needed (e.g. when starting anticoagulant therapy). It is used to depress clotting during the first 36 hrs of anticoagulant therapy (with or without warfarin therapy). Important uses of heparin include the following:

1 Prevention (especially during the peri-operative period) and treatment of *DVT*.
2 Prevention and treatment of *pulmonary embolism*.
3 *CVS*:
   a Atrial fibrillation (to prevent thrombus formation in atria and possible embolism).

    b Acute MI (in combination with thrombolytics).

    c Coronary angioplasty and placement of coronary stents (in combination with glycoprotein IIb/IIIa inhibitors).

4 *CNS*:
- CVA.

5 *Renal*:
- Haemodialysis/peritoneal dialysis.

6 *Anticoagulation during pregnancy*: Since heparin does not cross the placenta, if anti-coagulation is required during pregnancy due to any reason, heparin is the drug of choice. Warfarin, on the other hand, crosses placenta and is teratogenic and thus contraindicated during pregnancy.

7 *To preserve blood in vitro.*

Heparin: side effects

1 Commonest side effect is *bleeding*, especially with overdosage. *Protamine Sulphate 1% I/V* is the antidote for unfractionated heparin. However, it only partially reverses the effects of LMW heparins.

2 *Thrombocytopenia*: The mechanism is production of antibodies that bind to a complex of heparin and platelet factor IV. This side effect is usually seen with unfractionated heparin; it is less likely with LMW heparins.

3 *Osteoporosis* can occur with prolonged use. This in turn predisposes to spontaneous fractures.

4 *Transient alopecia.*

5 *Allergic reactions*: Asthma, urticaria and anaphylactic shock.

Warfarin: therapeutic uses

1 *Treatment of DVT and Pulmonary embolism.*

2 *CVS*:
- Acute MI.
- Atrial fibrillation.
- Artificial valve implantation.

3 *CNS*:
- CVA.

Mnemonic:
Warfarin: action, monitoring
WePT:
Warfarin works on the **e**xtrinsic pathway and is monitored by **PT**.

Warfarin: side effects

1 Commonest side effect is *bleeding*, especially with overdosage. Vit K I/V is the antidote.

2 *Teratogenicity*: Warfarin is contraindicated in pregnancy because it can cause bone defects and haemorrhages in the developing fetus.

3 Warfarin decreases the production of Protein C – an endogenous Vit K-dependent anticoagulant. Decreased production/deficiency of Protein C in turn may lead to the development of a period of *hypercoagulability* with subsequent dermal vascular necrosis early in the course of the therapy.

4 *Cytochrome P450-inducers* (e.g. barbiturates, carbamazapine, phenytoin) increase warfarin clearance and reduce its anticoagulant effect.

5 *Cytochrome P450-inhibitors* (e.g. amiodarone, SSRIs, cimetidine) reduce warfarin clearance and increase its anticoagulant effect.

Radioactive iodine I¹³¹ therapy: therapeutic uses

Thyrotoxicosis due to:

1 Graves' disease.

2 Toxic multi-nodular goitre.

3 Toxic nodule.

I¹³¹ is the only isotope used for the treatment of thyrotoxicosis; others are used for diagnosis. It is the drug of choice for the treatment of Graves' disease in patients <35 yrs of age (except in pregnant/lactating women, in whom it is contraindicated).

Hormonal contraceptives: therapeutic uses

1 Oral/parenteral/postcoital contraception.

2 Menstrual problems:

   a Severe dysmenorrhea ($\rightarrow \downarrow$ menstrual cramps).

   b Heavy menstrual bleeding.

   c Irregular periods ($\rightarrow$ regulates menstrual periods).

3 Hypogonadism and infertility (used both in females and males).

4 Hirsutism.

5 Acne.

6 Abortifacient.

7 Endometriosis.

8 Decreases the risk of breast CA, benign breast disease, endometrial CA, ovarian CA, ovarian cyst, pelvic inflammatory disease, ectopic pregnancy, iron-deficiency anaemia and rheumatoid arthritis.

9 Prostate: benign prostatic hypertrophy; CA prostate.

10 Osteoporosis in postmenopausal women.

11 For anabolic protein synthesis (used by athletes).

Hormonal contraceptives: side effects

1 *Severe*:

- *Vascular disorders*: Thromboembolic diseases, e.g. MI, stroke, DVT, pulmonary embolism. It is primarily caused by oestrogen.
- *Cancer (breast CA; endometrial CA)*: This side effect is also primarily caused by oestrogen. Combined use of progesterone decreases the probability of development of malignancy.
- *GIT*:

   a Cholestatic jaundice in patients taking progestin-containing drugs.

   b Hepatic adenomas.

   c Ischaemic bowel disease secondary to thrombosis of celiac and superior and inferior mesenteric arteries and veins.

- Depression.
- Skin: Alopecia, erythema multiforme (EM) and erythema nodosum (EN).

2 *Moderate*:

- *Break-through bleeding*: This side effect is seen both with combined and progestin-only pills especially during the first few months of the therapy.
- *Preparations containing androgenic progestins* can cause acne, increased skin pigmentation (especially in dark-skinned women), hirsutism, weight gain, ureteral dilation (similar to that observed during pregnancy), bacteriuria, vaginal infections and amenorrhea.

3 *Mild*:
- Mild and often transient headache.
- Worsening of migraine. It is often associated with an increased frequency of cerebrovascular accidents.
- Nausea, mastalgia, breakthrough bleeding and oedema. These side effects are related to the amount of oestrogen in the preparation (higher the amount, more chances of these side effects).
- Withdrawal bleeding sometimes fails to occur (most often with combination preparations) and may cause confusion with regards to pregnancy.
- Coadministration with potent inducers of hepatic microsomal metabolising enzymes (cytochrome P450) such as rifampicin may increase liver catabolism of oestrogens and progestins, thus diminishing the efficacy of oral contraceptives.

Hormonal contraceptives: contraindications

1 These drugs are contraindicated in patients with thrombophlebitis, thromboembolic phenomenon, cardiovascular and cerebrovascular disorders or a past history of these conditions.

2 They should not be used to treat vaginal bleeding when the cause is not known.

3 They should be avoided in patients with known or suspected tumours of breast or other oestrogen-dependent neoplasms.

4 Since these preparations cause aggravation of pre-existing disorders, they should be avoided or used with caution in patients with liver disease, diabetes, hypertension, asthma, eczema, optic neuritis, retrobulbar neuritis, migraine or convulsive disorders.

5 Since oral contraceptives can produce oedema, they should be used with caution in patients with heart failure or in whom oedema is otherwise undesirable or dangerous.

6 Since oestrogens may cause increase in the rate of growth of fibrinoids, drugs containing smallest amounts of oestrogen and mostly androgenic progestins should be selected in such cases.

7 They are contraindicated in adolescents in whom epiphyseal closure has not yet been completed.

Glucocorticoids: therapeutic uses

1 *Adrenal disorders*:
- a *Replacement therapy* for primary (Addison's disease)/secondary/tertiary-adrenocortical insufficiency: Glucocorticoids are life saving in these conditions.
- b Certain types of congenital adrenal hyperplasia (CAH) in which synthesis of some abnormal forms of glucocorticoids is stimulated by ACTH. In these conditions, exogenous administration of glucocorticoids suppresses the

endogenous release of ACTH, in turn suppressing the synthesis of abnormal forms of glucocorticoids.

c Differential diagnosis of Cushing's syndrome.

2 *Non-adrenal disorders*:

a Many *inflammatory/immunologic disorders*, e.g. asthma, connective tissue disorders (like SLE, rheumatoid arthritis, etc.), exophthalmos and organ transplantation.

b *Malignancies*: Hematopoietic cancers and chemotherapy-induced vomiting.

c *Neurologic disorders*: Multiple sclerosis.

d *Pregnancy*: Betamethasone is given to pregnant women in preterm labour. The aim is to hasten lung maturity of the preterm fetus. If not given, preterm neonate can die because of hypoxia.

e *Gram-negative bacteremia*.

f Raised ICP.

Glucocorticoids: side effects

1 *Iatrogenic Cushing's syndrome* and suppression of patients own capacity to synthesise glucocorticoids via a negative feedback effect on pituitary ACTH release.

2 *Secondary diabetes mellitus* due to hyperglycemia and increased glycogen storage.

3 *Secondary hypertension* due to increased mineralocorticoid activity (Na^+ and water retention).

4 Increased protein breakdown leading to *muscle wasting*.

5 Increased lipolysis and characteristic redistribution of fat leading to *moon face* and *buffalo hump* (at the back of the neck).

6 *Osteoporosis* due to increased activity of osteoclasts.

7 *Skin*: Acne, facial plethora, hirsutism, abdominal striae (purple-coloured).

8 *Proximal myopathy*.

9 *Suppression of growth in children*.

10 Suppression of inflammatory/immunological responses and T- and B-cell functions leading to *delayed wound healing* and *spread of infections*.

11 *Peptic ulceration*.

12 *Ocular*: Cataract and glaucoma.

13 *Menstrual disturbances*.

14 Precipitation of *psychotic episodes* like euphoria and depression.

CUSHINGS BAD MD:

Cataracts
Up all night (sleep disturbances)
Suppression of HPA axis
Hypertension/buffalo **H**ump
Infections
Necrosis (avascular)
Gain weight
Striae
Bone loss (osteoporosis)
Acne
Diabetes
Myopathy, moon faces
Depression and emotional changes

Aspirin: therapeutic uses

1 Three therapeutic dose ranges:
   a <300 mg/day: in this dose range aspirin is used as an antiplatelet agent.
   b 300–2400 mg/day: in this dose range aspirin is used as an antipyretic agent and analgesic.
   c 2400–4000 mg/day: in this dose range aspirin is used as an anti-inflammatory and uricosuric agent.
2 In neonates: Patent Ductus Arteriosus (PDA) closure after birth.
3 In females: to treat dysmenorrhea.
4 Prevention of familial polyposis coli (FPC)/CA colon.
5 Bartter's syndrome.
6 Niacin-induced cutaneous flushing (by inhibiting PGD_2).
7 Systemic mastocytosis.

Aspirin: side effects

1 *GIT*: Commonest side effect = peptic ulceration (gastric/duodenal). Complications of peptic ulcers include upper GI haemorrhage, perforation ($\rightarrow$ peritonitis) and gastric-outlet obstruction (due to excessive fibrosis). Aspirin-induced hypoprothrombinemia can also cause bleeding.
2 *Kidneys*: are often affected, by regular administration of aspirin. Important effects on kidneys include acute renal failure and interstitial nephritis.
3 *Lungs*: Aspirin can precipitate an acute attack of bronchial asthma in patients who are hypersensitive to this drug (especially those who are concomitantly suffering from nasal polyps). The mechanism is decreased synthesis of PGs and increased synthesis of leukotrienes ($\rightarrow$ bronchoconstriction).
4 *Toxicity: Salicylism*:
   • If taken in large doses, aspirin can cause tinnitus, deafness, vertigo, hyperventilation and respiratory acidosis.
   • At still higher doses, aspirin can cause metabolic acidosis, hyperpyrexia, dehydration, CV collapse, coma, convulsions and death.
5 *Reye's syndrome in children*: If aspirin is given to children with viral infections, they can develop Reye's syndrome (hepatic fatty degeneration $\rightarrow$ encephalopathy).
6 *Premature closure of PDA.*
7 *Prolongation of labour.*

ASPIRIN:

Asthma
Salicylism
Peptic ulcer disease/**P**hosphorylation-oxidation uncoupling/**PPH**/**P**latelet disaggregation/**P**remature closure of PDA
Intestinal blood loss
Reye's syndrome
Idiosyncracy
Noise (tinnitus)

Colchicine: therapeutic uses

1 Treatment of an *acute attack of Gout arthritis*.
2 Colchicine (in low doses) is used to prevent *recurrent attacks of Gouty arthritis*.

3 Prevention of attacks of *acute Mediterranean fever*.
4 *Psoriasis*.
5 *Primary biliary cirrhosis*.
6 *Sarcoid arthritis*.

Colchicine: side effects
1 Colchicine can severely damage liver and kidneys; overdosage (often fatal) must therefore be avoided.
2 NVD, abdominal pain, burning throat and haemorrhagic gastroenteritis (on oral administration).
3 Bone marrow suppression.
4 Peripheral neuritis and ascending CNS depression.
5 Myopathy and muscular paralysis.
6 Azoospermia.
7 Nephrotoxicity and extensive vascular damage.
8 Hair loss.

Morphine: therapeutic uses
1 Relief of severe *pain*: It also relieves the emotional and sensory aspects of pain. It can be given orally, parenterally (I/V/I/M) and via epidural and transdermal route.
2 Relief of *anxiety*.
3 *Left ventricular failure (LVF)*, with massive pulmonary oedema.
4 *Pre-anaesthetic* and *intra-operative medication*.
5 Terminal care of cancer patients.
6 *Antitussive* (cough reflex suppressed by an unknown mechanism).
7 *Antidiarrhoeal* (opioid receptors in the enteric nervous system stimulated → ↓ intestinal peristalsis). Constipation is a commonly known side effect of opioids.

Morphine: side effects
SCRAM:
Synergistic CNS depression with other drugs
Constipation
Respiratory depression
Addiction
Miosis

Morphine: pharmacological effects
MORPHINES:
Miosis
Orthostatic hypotension and bradycardia
Respiratory depression
Pain suppression
Histamine release/**H**ormonal alterations
Increased smooth muscle activity (biliary tract constriction)
Nausea
Euphoria
Sedation

Morphine: effects at mu receptor

PEAR:

Physical dependence

Euphoria

Analgesia

Respiratory depression

Naloxone: therapeutic uses

1 Antidote for acute opioid poisoning. There are multiple causes of coma with respiratory depression; opioid poisoning being one of them. If respiratory depression is d/t opioid poisoning, Nalaxone administration will rapidly reverse it thus differentiating coma with respiratory depression d/t opioid poisoning from other causes.

2 To diagnose a case of opioid addict.

3 Shock.

The **Na**rcotic **A**ntagonists are **NA**loxone and **NA**ltrexone.

Local anaesthetics: therapeutic uses

1 Surface anaesthesia (drops and sprays for eye, ear and laryngeal anaesthesia).

2 Infiltration anaesthesia.

3 Spinal anaesthesia (into the subarachnoid space).

4 Epidural anaesthesia (for painless child birth).

5 Nerve blocks (e.g. brachial plexus block).

6 As an analgesics (in malignancy).

7 As an anti-arrhythmic (lignocaine I/V for ventricular tachycardia).

Local anaesthetics: side effects

1 *CNS*: All local anaesthetists are capable of producing CNS side effects, most importantly, tonic-clonic convulsions, respiratory and cardiovascular depression and coma. These side effects are treated with diazepam or a short acting barbiturate such as thiopental; additionally, oxygen is given to prevent hypoxia. Occasionally, in non-responding cases, a neuromuscular blocking agent can be used to alleviate convulsions.

2 *CVS*:

  a With the exception of cocaine (a vasoconstrictor), all local anaesthetists are vasodilators. Thus they can cause hypotension, especially when given intravenously.

  b Cocaine, being a vasoconstrictor, can produce MI (due to coronary vasoconstriction), hypertension (due to systemic vasoconstriction) and cerebral haemorrhage.

  c Local anaesthetists can also produce heart blocks and other arrhythmias. Local anaesthetist, most notorious for its cardiovascular toxicity, is bupivacaine. When given intravenously, it can cause both hypotension and cardiac arrhythmias. It is difficult to treat cardiovascular toxicity of bupivacaine.

3 *Local neurotoxic effect*: Local anaesthetists when injected locally may cause permanent damage to the nerves of that area.

4 *Side effects caused by metabolites*: Metabolites of prilocaine are known to cause methemoglobinemia.

5 *Allergic manifestations*: include allergic dermatitis, asthmatic attack or severe fatal anaphylactic reaction.

Lignocaine: therapeutic uses
1 MI.
2 Digitalis intoxication.
3 Ventricular tachycardia.
4 As a local anaesthetic.
5 Open heart surgery.

Sedatives/hypnotics/benzodiazepines/barbiturates: therapeutic uses
1 *Relief of anxiety*: Buspirone produces anxiolytic effect without inducing sedation. It takes 1 week to produce full therapeutic effect. It is most commonly used to treat generalised anxiety in patients with a history of substance abuse.
2 *Relief of panic and phobic disorders*: Alprazolam and clonazepam are more efficacious than other benzodiazepines in treating panic and phobic disorders (neophobia/agoraphobia).
3 *Insomnia*: To induce and maintain sleep.
4 Pre-anaesthetic medication, induction and maintenance of anaesthesia: Thiopental is commonly used for the induction of anaesthesia. Benzodiazepines (like diazepam and midazolam) are used for sedation and amnesia before medical/surgical procedures.
5 *Epilepsy*: Phenobarbitone is often used as an anti-epileptic.
6 *Muscle spasm*: Diazepam is often used as a muscle relaxant.
7 *Ethanol and sedative/hypnotic withdrawal states*: Long-acting drugs like diazepam and chlordiazepoxide are used in these states.
8 *Psychiatric disorders* (like depression for short periods of time).

Benzodiazepines: antidote
'**Ben**ish is **off** with the **flu**':
Benzodiazepine effects **off** with **Flu**mazenil.

Benzodiazepines: pharmacological actions
'**Ben SCAM**s Sara into seduction **not by brain** but by muscle':
Sedation
anti**C**onvulsant
anti-**A**nxiety
Muscle relaxant
Not by brain: No antipsychotic activity.

Benzodiazepines: ones not metabolised by the liver (safe to use in liver failure)
'**O**utside **T**he **L**iver':
Oxazepam
Temazepam
Lorazepam
These undergo extrahepatic metabolism and do not form active metabolites.

Respiratory depression inducing drugs
'**STOP** breathing':
Sedatives and hypnotics
Trimethoprim
Opiates
Polymyxins

Lithium: therapeutic uses

1 In *manic-depressive (bipolar) illness* as a mood stabilising agent. Since lithium has a slow onset of action, neuroleptic and/or benzodiazepines are given at the beginning of lithium therapy. During the course of the therapy, antidepressants are often used concomitantly.
2 *Alcoholism* in manic-depressive patients.
3 *Mania*: Lithium is often used as an adjunct to antipsychotic therapy in this condition.
4 *Recurrent endogenous depression*: In this condition, lithium is used as an adjunct to TCAs or SSRI therapy.
5 *Schizophrenia/schizoaffective disorders.*
6 *Syndrome of inappropriate ADH secretion (SIADH)*: Lithium is an ADH antagonist and thus can be used in SIADH, although demeclocycline is the drug of choice.

Lithium: side effects

1 *CNS*: Tremors, choreoathetosis, ataxia, increased motor activity, mental confusion, dysarthria and aphasia.
2 *GIT*: N, V, D and anorexia (it is of central origin).
3 *Renal*:
   a Loss of ability of collecting tubules to conserve water (under the influence of ADH) → excessive free water clearance → polyuria and polydypsia. This is called nephrogenic diabetes insipidus.
   b Chronic interstitial nephritis.
   c Minimal change glomerulonephritis (→ nephrotic syndrome).
4 *Thyroid*: Hypothyroidism and enlargement of thyroid gland.
5 *CVS*: Brady- and tachycardia (called 'sick sinus syndrome') and T-wave flattening.
6 *Use in pregnancy*: Teratogenic.
7 *Use in infants*: Poor suck and Moro's reflexes (i.e. ↓ motor activity), hypothermia, hepatomegaly, Na^+ retention (→ oedema; weight gain).
8 *Miscellaneous*: Transient acneiform eruptions, folliculitis, leukocytosis, etc.

LITH:
Leukocytosis
Insipidus (diabetes insipidus, tied to polyuria)
Tremors/**T**eratogenesis
Hypothyroidism

Monoamine oxidase inhibitors (MAOIs): side effects

Restlessness, insomnia, excitement, convulsions, throbbing headache, drowsiness, postural hypotension, atropine-like side effects, weight gain due to an increase in appetite, sexual dysfunctions (impotence) and cheese reaction.

Cheese reaction: Normally, when tyramine containing food stuffs (like cheese, yoghurt, broad beans, red wine, etc.) are taken, tyramine is broken down by intestinal and hepatic monoamine oxidase enzymes (MAO-A and MAO-B). However, on MAOIs administration, MAO enzymes are inhibited so that tyramine is not destroyed and it reaches the systemic circulation. From there, it is actively taken up by the noradrenergic nerve terminals where it displaces noradrenaline from its receptor sites causing marked increase in the intraneuronal concentrations of noradrenaline. This in turn causes spontaneous leakage of increased amounts of noradrenaline into the synaptic cleft that may lead to hypertensive crisis, intracranial haemorrhage, epistaxis or throbbing headache.

Carbamazepine: therapeutic uses

1 It is the drug of choice for partial seizures especially temporal lobe epilepsy.
2 Grand mal epilepsy.
3 Trigeminal neuralgia.
4 Bipolar disorder (mania).

Sodium valproate: therapeutic uses

1 *Epilepsy*: Grand mal, petit mal, mixed grand mal-petit mal, absence seizures, partial seizures, secondary generalised tonic clonic seizures, akinetic epilepsy, atonic epilepsy, myoclonic jerks and infantile spasms.
2 *Resistant manic-depressive (bipolar) illness.*

Sodium valproate: side effects
VALPROATE:
Vomiting
Alopecia
Liver toxicity
Pancreatitis/Pancytopenia
Retention of fats (weight gain)
Edema (peripheral oedema)
Appetite increase
Tremor
Enzyme inducer (liver)

Levodopa: therapeutic uses

1 *Parkinsonism*: Levodopa particularly ameliorates bradykinesia. However, it is not curative and responsiveness decreases with time.
2 *Galactorrhea/hyperprolactinemia.*

Bromocriptine: therapeutic uses

1 *Treatment of Parkinsonism in combination with L-dopa*: Bromocriptine is not effective in drug-induced extra-pyramidal symptoms.

Dose:
- 1st week: 1–1.25 mg at night.
- 2nd week: 2–2.5 mg at night.
- 3rd week: 2.5 mg twice a day.
- 4th week: 2.5 mg three times a day.
- Usual therapeutic range 10–30 mg/day in divided doses.

2 *For prevention and suppression of lactation in mothers.*

3 Treatment of *prolactin-secreting pituitary tumour* and associated hypogonadism, galactorrhea and infertility.

4 Treatment of *growth hormone-secreting pituitary tumour* (acromegaly). Physiologically, dopamine inhibits the release of growth hormone.

Bromocriptine: side effects

1 *GIT*: N, V and anorexia.

2 *CVS*: Postural hypotension, tachycardia and cardiac arrhythmias.

3 *CNS*:
   a Dyskinesias with abnormal movements. It is also seen with levodopa. These can be reversed by simply decreasing the dose.
   b Behavioural effects: Confusion, hallucinations and delusions. As compared to levodopa, behavioural effects are more common with bromocriptine. Both levodopa and bromocriptine are contraindicated in patients with a history of psychosis.

4 *Ergot-related side effects*: include pulmonary infiltrates and erythromelalgia (red, swollen and tender feet and hands).

Imipramine: therapeutic uses

1 *Depression*: It is particularly useful in depressed patients with sleep disturbances, poor appetite and weight loss.

2 *Neurosis* associated with depression.

3 *Nocturnal enuresis* and *attention-deficit hyperkinetic syndrome* in children.

4 *Pain*:
   a Unexplained chronic body pains.
   b Neuralgias (trigeminal/hypoglossal/herpetic neuralgias).

5 *Panic and phobic disorders.*

6 *Alcoholism.*

7 *Obsessive compulsive disorders* (antipsychotic and antidepressant drugs are given in combination).

8 *Manic-depressive (bipolar) disorder.*

Tricyclic antidepressants (TCA): side effects

1 *Anticholinergic*: Blurring of vision, photophobia, dryness of mouth, metabolic or sour- taste, tachycardia, constipation, and urinary retention.

2 *Cerebral toxicity*: Sedation, lethargy, delirium, confusion, excitement, convulsions, increased frequency of epileptic fits and ataxia.

3 *Cardiotoxicity*: Arrhythmias like AV extrasystole, ventricular tachycardia (VT) and ventricular fibrillation (VF), MI.

4 *Hypersensitivity/allergic manifestations*: Skin rash, agranulocytosis, photosensitivity, cholestatic jaundice and tremors.

TCAS:
Thrombocytopenia
Cardiac (arrhythmia like AV extrasystole, VT, VF, MI)
Anticholinergic
Seizures

Benzylpenicillin: therapeutic uses

1 Beta-hemolytic streptococcal infections (acute tonsillitis, pharyngitis, skin and bone infections).
2 Staphylococcal infections (only non-beta lactamase producing strains).
3 Pneumocccal infections (pneumocccal pneumonia/meningitis).
4 Meningococcal meningitis (causative organism: *Neisseria menigititis*).
5 Gonococcal urethritis (causative organism: *Neisseria gonorrhea*).
6 Syphilis (causative organism: *Treponema pallidum*).
7 Anaerobic infections above the diaphragm.
8 Actinomycosis.
9 Anthrax.
10 Erysipeloid.
11 Fusospirochetal diseases (like Torch mouth, Vincent's angina).
12 Leptospirosis.
13 Listeriosis.
14 Pasteurella multocida-induced diseases.

Benzylpenicillin: side effects

1 *Allergic reactions* include:
  a Urticaria, severe pruritus and joint swelling.
  b Skin rashes of various types.
  c Serum sickness-like syndrome.
  d Allergic renal disturbances (interstitial nephritis).
  e Allergic blood dyscrasias (hemolytic anaemia).
  f Acute anaphylactic shock.
2 *Jarisch-Herxhimier reaction*: In cases of syphilis, large amounts of toxins and antigens are released when first dose of benzylpenicillin kills the causative organism (treponema pallidum). These toxins and antigens in turn cause worsening of the symptoms (increase in the size of the lesions, malaise and joint pains). This is called Jarisch-Herxhimier reaction.
3 *Hyperkalemia and hypernatremia* in large doses.
4 *Superadded infection*: On oral administration of large doses of benzylpenicillin, these drugs kill normal bacterial flora of the body. This in turn causes growth of opportunistic organisms (e.g. candida albicans, *Clostridium difficile*, etc.) and may result in superadded infections e.g. pseudomembranous colitis caused by clostridium difficile (treated by metronidazole and vancomycin).

Cephalosporins: therapeutic uses

1 *1st Generation*:
  • UTI.
  • Surgical prophylaxis.
  • Minor staphylococcal infections (cellulitis/soft tissue abscesses).

2 *2nd Generation*:
- *H. Influenzae* infection.
- *Morexella catarrhalis* infection.
- Sinusitis.
- Otitis media.
- Meningitis.
- Anaerobic (*Bacteroides fragilis*) infection.
- Peritonitis.
- Diverticulitis.
- Surgical prophylaxis (colorectal surgery, hysterectomy, appendicectomy, etc.).

3 *3rd and 4th Generation*:
- Meningitis.
- Febrile neutropenic patients.
- Lyme's disease.
- Chancroid.
- Gonorrhea.

Cephalosporins: side effects

1 *Hypersensitivity reactions*: These include allergy, anaphylaxis, fever, hemolytic anaemia, granulocytopenia, nephritis and skin rash. Cross-allergy is seen between penicillins and cephalosporins in approximately 5–10% of the patients. Patients with a history of allergy to penicillins should not receive cephalosporins.

2 *Toxicity*: Local irritation with I/M injection; thrombophlebitis with I/V injection; renal toxicity like interstitial nephritis and tubular necrosis; hypoprothrombinemia; bleeding disorders (when ceftriaxone is administered in a dose of >02 gm/day for long periods); biliary sludging syndrome ($\rightarrow$ cholelithiasis); superadded infections.

Quinolones: therapeutic uses

1st Generation:

1 Uncomplicated UTI.

2 Resistant bacillary dysentery.

2nd Generation:

1 Respiratory tract infections (pneumonias).

2 Tuberculosis (as a Second-line agent).

3 Typhoid fever.

4 Bacterial diarrhoea (e.g. caused by shigella, salmonella, *E coli*, etc.).

5 UTI caused by pseudomonas; chlamydial and gonococcal prostatitis, urethritis and cervicitis.

6 Systemic pseudomonas infection.

7 Intrabdominal, soft tissue, bone and joint infections.

8 Eradication of meningococci from carriers.

9 Prophylactically in neutropenic patients.

Quinolones: side effects

1 *GIT*: N, V, D; hepatotoxicity.

2 *CVS*: Prolongation of QT interval.

3 *Endocrine*: Hyperglycemia (occurs with gatifloxacin).
4 *Joints*: Reversible arthropathy and tendonitis.
5 *Allergic reactions*: Photosensitivity.

Sulfonamides: therapeutic uses

1 As topical agents: sulfonamides are used in trachoma and bacterial conjunctivitis; also in burn cases, sulfonamides are used as a prophylaxis against superadded infections.
2 UTI.
3 Ulcerative colitis.
4 Enteritis.
5 Rheumatoid arthritis.
6 Dermatitis herpetiformis.
7 Pneumocystis carinii pneumonia (Co-tromixazole).
8 Resistant malaria (Fansidar – a combination of sulphadoxine + pyrimethamine).
9 Acute toxoplasmosis (Fansidar).

Co-tromixazole: therapeutic uses

1 Pneumocystis carinii pneumonia.
2 *H. influenzae.*
3 *Streptococcus pneumoniae.*
4 *Klebsiella pneumoniae.*
5 *Moraxella catarrhalis.*
6 Non-tuberculous mycobacterial infections.
7 GIT infections (like shigellosis, typhoid fever).
8 UTI.
9 Gonococcal urethritis.

Co-trimoxazole/sulfonamide: side effects

1 *Hyper-sensitivity reactions*:
  a *Common*: Fever and skin rash.
  b *Rare*: Exfoliative dermatitis, polyarteritis nodosa (PAN) and Stevens-Johnson syndrome (SJS).
2 *GIT*: N, V, D and elevation of hepatic aminotransferases.
3 *Hematotoxicity*: Hemolytic anaemia (especially in patients with G6PD deficiency), aplastic anaemia, granulocytopenia and thrombocytopenia.
4 *Nephrotoxicity*: Sulfonamides can precipitate in the acidic urine, in turn causing crystalluria and hematuria.
5 *Use in pregnancy*: When used in third trimester, sulfonamides, by displacing bilirubin from the plasma proteins, allow free bilirubin to cross BBB and get deposited in fetal brain causing kernicterus.
6 *Important drug interactions*: Sulfonamides compete with other drugs (like warfarin and methotrexate) for plasma protein binding. This in turn can transiently raise the levels of the said drugs.

Macrolides: therapeutic uses

1 Alternative to penicillins in patients who are penicillin allergic/resistant.
2 Atypical pneumonia due to mycoplasma pneumoniae and legionella.

3 *Campylobacter jejuni* infections.
4 Chlamydial infections (UTI, trachoma, psittacosis).
5 Diphtheria (caused by *Corynebacterium diphtheriae*).
6 Whooping cough.
7 Toxoplasmosis.

Macrolides: side effects

1 *GIT*: When taken empty stomach, they can cause epigastric distress, NVD and abdominal pain by stimulating motilin receptors.
2 *Cholestatic jaundice*: It occurs with erythromycin estolate, especially when used in pregnant ladies.
3 *Drug interactions*: Both erythromycin and clarithromycin inhibit hepatic cytochrome P450 → ↓ metabolism of drugs being metabolised by this enzymatic system (e.g. anticoagulants, carbamazapine, digoxin and theophylline) → ↑ side effects. Azithromycin (because of its lactone ring structure) does not inhibit hepatic cytochrome P450 and thus it is free of above mentioned drug interactions.
4 *Blood dyscrasias*: Eosinophilia and leukocytosis.
5 *Allergic reactions*: Fever and skin rash.
6 Intravenous administration can cause *thrombophlebitis*.

Amoebicides: therapeutic uses

1 Amoebiasis d/t *Entamoeba histolytica* (both intestinal and hepatic).
2 Giardiasis.
3 *H. pylori* eradication.
4 Trichomoniasis (both vaginal and urethral).
5 Acute ulcerative gingivitis.
6 Anaerobic infections (d/t *Bacteroides fragilis*).
7 Abdominal surgery.
8 Clostridial infection (like pseudomembranous colitis).
9 Brain abscess.
10 Indolent ulcers.
11 Rosacea.

Amoebicides: side effects

If given for 3–5 days, only a few and mild side effects develop. Severe side effects only develop when amoebicides are given for up to 10 days.

1 At injection site, pain, tenderness, muscle weakness and abscess formation can occur.
2 Cardiotoxicity in the form of arrhythmias and CCF is rare.
3 N, V (of central origin) and D.
4 Generalised muscle weakness associated with tenderness, stiffness, tremors and mild paresthesias.

Atropine: therapeutic uses

1 *Before and during surgery*:
   • *Before surgery/pre-anaesthetic medication*: Almost half an hour before administering GA, atropine is given to prevent laryngeal spasm because it extensively decreases tracheobronchial secretions.

- *During surgery*: To prevent reflex slowing or asystole due to handling of viscera in abdominal surgery.

2 *Motion sickness*: It is given prophylactically before travelling because it has its effect on vestibular pathway.

3 *Parkinsonism*: It is used to counteract excessive ACh effect when there is less dopamine.

4 *Ophthalmic Uses*:
- To dilate pupil.
- To give rest to the eye in inflammatory conditions (nowadays adrenergic drugs are preferred for giving rest to eye).
- For measuring refractive error in children and in non-cooperative patients.
- For breaking adhesions in anterior and posterior synechiae. In such cases, atropine is given alternatively with miotics.

5 *Treatment of organophosphorous compound and mushroom poisoning.*

6 *Antispasmodic for treating colicky abdominal pain.*

7 *Antidiarrhoeal*: It relaxes smooth muscles.

8 *Antisialagogue*: It reduces salivary secretions.

9 *Bronchial asthma*: It causes bronchodilatation.

10 *Nocturnal enuresis (bed-wetting) in children.*

11 *Hyperhydrosis (excessive sweating).*

12 *Treatment of bradycardia*: In acute MI, hyperactive carotid sinus reflex and tight-collar syndrome.

Atropine: side effects

1 *Hyperthermia ('atropine fever')*: inhibition of sweating $\rightarrow \downarrow$ heat loss from the body $\rightarrow$ fever. This is the most dangerous side effect of antimuscarinic drugs and is potentially fatal especially in infants. Atropine is relatively contraindicated in infants because of the danger of hyperthermia.

2 *'Atropine flush'*: At toxic doses, atropine can cause dilatation of the subcutaneous blood vessels causing the skin to appear 'red'. This is called 'atropine flush' and is the diagnostic sign of toxicity with antimuscarinic drugs.

3 *'Atropine madness'*: At toxic doses, atropine can cause delirium, convulsions and hallucinations – called atropine madness. Central muscarinic receptors are probably involved.

4 *Pupillary dilatation* $\rightarrow$ blurring of vision. Pupillary dilatation can also precipitate an acute attack of angle-closure glaucoma (atropine is relatively contraindicated in patients of angle-closure glaucoma).

5 *Dryness of mouth* (d/t inhibition of salivation).

6 *Tachycardia* $\rightarrow$ tachyarrhythmias may occur. At toxic doses, atropine can cause a paradoxical effect (i.e. blockade of intra-ventricular conduction).

7 *Constipation.*

8 *Urinary retention*, especially in elderly men with BPH. Atropine is relatively contraindicated in patients with BPH.

Pilocarpine: therapeutic uses

- For treatment of glaucoma (both closed-angle and wide-angle).
- To reduce the effect of mydriatics, e.g. atropine, homatropine and eucatropine.
- For the treatment of inflammatory conditions of the eye.

- To break the adhesions b/w iris and lens (posterior synechiae) or iris and cornea (anterior synechiae). In such cases, it is used alternatively with mydriatics.
- In patients of Parkinsonism being treated with anticholinergic drugs like benzhexol.
- Xerostomia.
- Sjögren's syndrome.
- Patients undergoing radiotherapy.

Note: It is not used for systemic diseases because it may lead to increase in tracheo-bronchial secretions and pulmonary oedema.

Physostigmine: therapeutic uses

1 Ophthalmic uses:
  a Acute congestive glaucoma: Physostigmine and pilocarpine eye drops plus acetazolamide (orally or by injection) are used for the treatment of acute congestive glaucoma. Just like pilocarpine, physostigmine lowers the IOP by improving the drainage of aqueous humour by its miotic effect.
  b To counteract the mydriatics effect of homatropine.
  c To break the adhesions b/w lens and iris or iris and cornea (known as posterior and anterior synechiae, respectively). In such cases, it is used alternatively with the mydriatics like homatropine.
2 It is the drug of first choice in cases of atropine poisoning. It is also recommended in cases of phenothiazines, antihistamines and TCA poisoning. Physostigmine being a tertiary amine can cross the BBB and reverse the toxic CNS effects of these drugs. Neostigmine, on the other hand, cannot do the same because being a quaternary amine, it cannot cross the BBB.
3 Physostigmine can be of some help in patients of senile dementia and Alzheimer's disease where there is deficiency of ACh in CNS due to loss of cholinergic neurons in memory pathway (septohippocampal pathway). If, however, physostigmine is given in very high doses, it can cause death by respiratory failure.

Neostigmine: therapeutic uses

1 Relief of abdominal distension/paralytic ileus.
2 Relief of urinary retention in bladder atonia.
3 Relief of myasthenia gravis.

Differeces between Physostigmine and Neostigmine

LMNOP:

Lipid soluble
Miotic
Natural
Orally absorbed well
Physostigmine

Neostigmine, on the contrary, is:
- Water soluble
- Used in myasthenia gravis

- Synthetic
- Poor oral absorption

Neuromuscular (NM) blocking agents: therapeutic uses
1 As adjuvant to anaesthesia.
2 For rapid endotracheal intubation (suxamethonium is used).
3 In crush injuries of chest (to provide rest to the respiratory muscles).
4 With electroconvulsive therapy (ECT) in cases of severe depression (to prevent trauma).
5 For diagnosis of myasthenia gravis.
6 Treatment of poisoning due to convulsant drugs, e.g. strychnine.
7 For treatment of tetanus and status epilepticus.

Suxamethonium: therapeutic uses
1 For rapid endotracheal intubation.
2 Short procedures (e.g. local surgeries, upper or lower GI endoscopy, ECT, etc.).

Acetazolamide: therapeutic uses
1 Rarely used as a diuretic (limited efficacy).
2 Glaucoma.
3 Prevention and treatment of mountain sickness.
4 Familial periodic paralysis.
5 Petit-mal epilepsy.
6 Correction of metabolic alkalosis (especially diuretics-induced).

Beta blockers: therapeutic uses
1 *CVS*:
   a Antihypertensive (beta blockers → ↓ cardiac output and ↓ renin secretion).
   b Anti-arrhythmic.
   c Ischaemic heart disease (angina and MI).
   d Chronic (not acute) heart failure: Beta blockers have been proved to reduce mortality in heart failure cases by some unknown mechanism.
   e Hypertrophic obstructive cardiomyopathy (HOCM).
2 *CNS*:
   a Migraine prophylaxis.
   b Familial tremors.
   c Anxiety-related tremors.
3 *Thyroid*: Thyrotoxicosis (Graves' disease) and thyroid crisis.
4 *Eye*: Glaucoma (β-blockers → ↓ secretion of aqueous humour).
5 *Abdomen*:
   a Portal hypertension.
   b Pheochromocytoma: Treated by combined α and β-blocking agent (e.g. labetalol).

Beta blockers: side effects
1 *CNS*:
- Insomnia, bad dreams, lassitude and depression. Beta blockers with low lipid-solubility and thus poor CNS penetration (e.g. atenolol, nadolol) produce only minimal CNS side effects.

2 *CVS*:
- Because of negative inotropic and chronotropic effects, β-blockers can cause bradycardia, AV block and CCF.

3 *Respiratory system*:
- By causing bronchoconstriction, β-blockers can precipitate an acute attack of asthma/COPD.

4 *Metabolic*:
- In case a diabetic develops hypoglycemia, the symptoms of hypoglycemia will be masked by β-blockers. Hypoglycemia induces sympathomimetic symptoms (like anxiety, tremors, palpitations, etc.), which will be masked by β-blockers. Thus hypoglycemia may go unnoticed. β-blockers also decrease glucose mobilisation from the liver leading to further worsening of hypoglycemia. Untreated hypoglycemia can cause permanent brain damage. Because of this reason β-blockers are relatively contraindicated in diabetes mellitus.

5 *Sexual disturbances*:
- Erectile dysfunction in males.

6 *Peripheries*:
- Coolness and fatigue of extremities d/t decreased blood flow to skeletal muscles.

7 *Oculo-mucocutaneous syndrome*:
- Characterised by skin rash (psoriasis), dryness of conjunctiva, corneal ulcers and ulceration of nasal mucosa.

Beta-blockers: side effects
'**BBC** **L**ost **V**iewership **I**n **R**awalpindi':
Bradycardia
Bronchoconstriction
Claudication
Lipids
Vivid dreams and nightmares
–ve **I**notropic action
Reduced sensitivity to hypoglycemia

Beta-blockers: main contraindications, cautions
ABCDE:
Asthma
Block (heart block)
COPD
Diabetes mellitus
Electrolyte (hyperkalemia)

Alpha adrenergic blockers: therapeutic uses
Non-selective alpha-antagonists

1 *Hypertension*:
- a Essential hypertension.
- b Many drugs of abuse (e.g. amphetamine, cocaine, etc.) can cause severe hypertension. Alpha-antagonists by causing vasodilatation can effectively treat this drug-induced hypertension.
- c Sudden cessation of clonidine can cause rebound hypertension. This

phenomenon can be treated with phentolamine.

2 *Pheochromocytoma*: Phenoxybenzamine is the drug of choice.

3 *Carcinoid syndrome* (secretes serotonin): Phenoxybenzamine blocks serotonin receptors.

4 *Mastocytosis*: Phenoxybenzamine blocks H_1 receptors.

5 *Accidental local infiltration of a potent α-agonist* (e.g. epinephrine) can cause tissue necrosis d/t vasoconstriction. Alpha-antagonists can reverse this action.

6 *Erectile dysfunction*: Phentolamine or yohimbine injection directly into the penis.

Selective alpha-antagonists (prazosin; doxazosin; terazosin)

1 Hypertension.

2 BPH.

Alpha adrenergic blockers: side effects

1 *Postural/orthostatic hypotension*, especially with the first dose. Therefore first dose is usually small and taken just before going to the bed.

2 *Reflex tachycardia*: In patients with coronary artery disease, angina may be pre-cipitated due to reflex tachycardia. Tachycardia is less severe with α1-selective blockers.

3 *N, V, D* due to parasympathetic dominance over the sympathetic discharge.

4 *Nasal stuffiness.*

5 *Sedation.*

6 *Failure/delayed/retrograde ejaculation.*

Methyldopa: therapeutic uses

1 *Hypertension*:

   a *Essential HTN*: The major compensatory response is Na^+ and water retention. The added advantage of methyldopa (as an antihypertensive agent) is that it can be used in late pregnancy as it does not produce toxic effects on mother and fetus.

   b *Hypertensive crisis*: 200–250 mg I/V; can be repeated after 6hrs.

   c Sudden discontinuation of methyldopa or clonidine should be avoided otherwise severe *rebound hypertension* can occur, which can either be treated by reinstituting methyldopa/clonidine therapy or by administering alpha-antagonists, e.g. phentolamine.

2 *Carcinoid syndrome*: is d/t carcinoid tumour of enterochromaffin cells in the intestine producing large amounts of serotonin, substance P, PGs and bradykinin. Serotonin causes increased GI motility with resultant diarrhoea. Methyldopa reduces serotonin formation.

Clonidine: therapeutic uses

1 HTN.

2 Alcohol/drug withdrawal.

Guanithidine: therapeutic uses

1 Used to treat moderate to severe hypertensive cases.

2 Autonomic hyperreflexia.

3 Ophthalmic uses: Glaucoma; Graves' disease (lid retraction and thyrotoxicosis).

Dantrolene: therapeutic uses

1 *Muscle spasms*: Certain CNS diseases (e.g. cerebral palsy, multiple sclerosis and stroke) are associated with abnormally high reflex activity in those neuronal pathways that control skeletal muscles. The result is painful muscle spasms. Dantrolene by reducing the release of calcium from the sarcoplasmic reticulum relieves such spasms.

2 *Malignant hyperthermia*: General anaesthetic agents (like succinylcholine and tubocurarine) can cause massive release of calcium from the sarcoplasmic reticulum of the skeletal muscles. Dantrolene, by reducing the release of calcium from the sarcoplasmic reticulum, is the drug of choice in this condition.

Adrenaline: therapeutic uses

1 *Emergency uses*:
  - Acute anaphylactic shock.
  - Cardiac resuscitation.
2 *Topical uses*:
  - Topical hemostasis.
  - Topical agent for glaucoma: Alpha agonists by inducing mydriasis reduce conjunctival itching.
3 *Use in anaesthesia*:
  - To prolong the actions of infiltration anaesthesia.

Adrenaline: side effects

1 It can produce *anxiety-related symptoms*, e.g. fears, restlessness, headache, tremors and palpitations.
2 *Cardiac arrhythmias*: Excessive sympathomimetic effect can precipitate arrhythmias.
3 *Coronary vasoconstriction*: It can precipitate angina pectoris or myocardial infarction.
4 *Tissue necrosis* (d/t intense vasoconstriction).
5 *Pulmonary oedema/haemorrhage*.
6 *Cerebral haemorrhage*.

Noradrenaline: therapeutic uses

1 Cardiogenic shock.
2 Oliguric patients.

Isoprenaline: therapeutic uses

1 Used as a bronchodilator.
2 Cardiac stimulant in heart blocks.
3 For maintenance of systolic BP in cardiogenic and septic shock.

Salbutamol: therapeutic uses

1 Bronchial asthma.
2 COPD.
3 To prevent premature labour (Ritodrine is preferred).

Alpha-1 agonists: therapeutic uses

1 *Nose*: As nasal decongestant.
2 *Eyes*: Alpha agonists (e.g. phenylephrine) by inducing mydriasis, reduce conjunctival itching. These drugs do not cause cycloplegia. Newer α_2-selective agonists (e.g. Apra-clonidine) reduce aqueous synthesis and are thus useful in the treatment of glaucoma.
3 *Hypotension*:
    a For treating spinal shock (α agonists $\rightarrow$ vasoconstriction $\rightarrow$ $\uparrow$ BP). Conversely, shock due to septicemia or MI is made worse by α agonists and thus they should be avoided in such cases.
    b Chronic orthostatic hypotension d/t inadequate sympathetic tone: Ephedrine or a new $\alpha 1$-agonist midodrine can be used.

Ephedrine: therapeutic uses

1 Nasal decongestant (causes constriction of nasal blood vessels). Nowadays alpha-1 selective agonists are used (like xylometazoline).
2 As mydriatics.
3 As presser agent in chronic orthostatic hypotension.
4 Urinary stress incontinence, especially in females because it contracts the detrusor muscle and relaxes the sphincter.
5 Bronchial asthma (causes bronchodilatation; given prophylactically). Beta-2 selective agonists are preferred nowadays.
6 Whooping cough (relieves the paroxysms).
7 Myasthenia gravis (stimulates NM transmission). It thus enhances the effect of neostigmine (an anticholinesterase).
8 In skin allergies (counteract the effects of histamine by causing vasoconstriction).

Ergot alkaloids: therapeutic uses

1 *Migraine*:
    a *Acute attack*: Ergotamine is used.
    b *Prevention*: Ergonovine and methysergide are used.
2 *Postpartum haemorrhage*: Ergotamine and ergonovine are used.

Migraine: prophylaxis drugs

'**V**ery **V**olatile **P**harmacotherapeutic **A**gents **F**or **M**igraine **P**rophylaxis':
Verapamil
Valproic acid
Pizotifen
Amitriptyline
Flunarizine
Methysergide
Propranolol

Digitalis: therapeutic uses

1 *CCF*: Digitalis $\rightarrow$ positive inotropic effect $\rightarrow$ $\uparrow$ force of cardiac contraction.
2 *Arrhythmias*:
    a Atrial fibrillation/flutter, associated with hypotension or pulmonary oedema. Digitalis decreases the ventricular rate by depressing SA node, decreasing the

AV nodal conduction (negative chronotropic effect) and improving cardiac contraction (positive inotropic effect).

b Paroxysmal atrial tachycardia.

c AV-nodal tachycardia.

Calcium channel blockers: therapeutic uses

1 *CVS*:

   a HTN.

   b Angina.

   c Supraventricular arrhythmias: Verapamil and diltiazem are used; nifedipine and other dihydropyridines are not used as anti-arrhythmics (nifedipine → ↓ B.P → reflex tachycardia → facilitates arrhythmias rather than suppressing them).

2 *CNS*:

   a Subarachnoid haemorrhage (SAH): Nimodipine is used.

   b Migraine prophylaxis.

3 *Raynaud's syndrome.*

4 *Preterm labour.*

Ace inhibitors: therapeutic uses

1 *CVS*:

- HTN (usually given with thiazide diuretics; can be given with β-blockers).
- MI.
- CCF.

2 *Diabetic Nephropathy.*

Captopril (an ACE inhibitor): side effects

CAPTOPRIL:

Cough

Angioedema/**A**granulocytosis

Proteinuria/**P**otassium excess

Taste changes

Orthostatic hypotension

Pregnancy contraindication/**P**ancreatitis/**P**ressure drop (first dose hypertension)

Renal failure (and renal artery stenosis contraindication)/**R**ash

Indomethacin inhibition

Leukopenia/**L**iver toxicity

Vasodilator drugs (hydralazine; minoxidil; Na nitroprusside): therapeutic uses

1 Hypertensive emergency.

Nitroglycerin: therapeutic uses

1 For prophylaxis and treatment of classical angina pectoris.

2 Treatment of variant/prinzmetal's (angiospastic) angina.

3 Treatment of unstable angina.

4 Cyanide poisoning.

Allopurinol: therapeutic uses

1 Primary and secondary hyperuricemia.
2 Chronic gout; chronic tophaceous gout; gouty nephropathy.
3 Prevention of deposition of urate crystals in tissues and occurrence of urate renal stones.
4 As an antiprotozoal agent.

Used in patients allergic or intolerant to probenecid and sulfinpyrazone.

Allopurinol: side effects

1 Exacerbation of an acute attack of gouty arthritis: In order to prevent these attacks, colchicine and indomethacin are given (before starting allopurinol therapy).
2 Hypersensitivity reactions: e.g. pruritic maculopapular lesions and exfoliative dermatitis.
3 Peripheral neuritis.
4 Necrotising vasculitis.
5 Bone marrow suppression.
6 Aplastic anaemia and cataract formation (rare).
7 N, V, D.

Insulin: side effects

1 *Hypoglycemia*: Brain damage may occur in turn. Prompt administration of glucose (sugar/candy by mouth, intravenous glucose or intramuscular glucagon) is the emergency treatment of hypoglycemia.
2 *Rebound hyperglycemia*: This can follow excessive insulin administration and results from the release of insulin-opposing hormones (glucagon, adrenaline, glucocorticoids, growth and thyroid hormones).
3 *Immunological complications*: Regular insulin administration can lead to the formation of antibodies against insulin or non-insulin protein contaminants. This in turn may cause insulin resistance or insulin allergy. Immunological complications primarily occur with bovine insulin and are uncommon with the currently available highly-purified human insulin.
4 *Lipodystrophy/lipohypertrophy* at the site of injection.

Chlorpromazine: therapeutic uses

A *Treatment of psychiatric patients*:
   1 Symptomatic treatment of schizophrenia.
   2 Organic psychosis.
   3 Manic episode and affective disorders.
B *Non-psychiatric indications*:
   1 Tourette's syndrome.
   2 Non-manic excited states.
   3 To control disturbed behaviour in Alzheimer's disease.
   4 Migraine.
   5 Alcoholic hallucinosis.
   6 Nausea and vomiting.
   7 Intractable hiccup.
   8 Persistent pruritus.

9 Pre-operative sedation.
10 To potentiate the effects of analgesics.

Chlorpromazine: side effects

1 *Neurological side effects*:
   a Extrapyramidal side effects (like Parkinsonism) – acute dystonias, akathisia, tardive dyskinesia, perioral tremors – also called Rabbit's syndrome.
   b Neuroleptic malignant syndrome.
2 *ANS side effects*: By blocking muscarinic receptors, atropine-like effects can develop, e.g. dryness of mouth, tachycardia, blurring of vision, etc.
3 *CVS side effects*:
   a α-1 receptor blockade results in decreased blood pressure, decreased resting heart rate, vasodilatation and decrease in peripheral resistance (→ orthostatic hypotension).
   b ECG changes like prolonged QT interval; prolonged PT interval; flattening or notching of P wave; ST segment depression; ventricular tachycardia (VT) – caused by local anaesthetic effect; quinidine-like effects.
4 *Hypothalamic and endocrine side effects*: By blocking α-1 receptors, ADH, oestrogen, progesterone, corticosteroids and growth hormone levels are decreased.
5 Drug interactions:
   a They have an additive effect with sedatives and hypnotics.
   b They increase the toxicity of H_1-antagonists, α-blockers and quinidine.
   c They increase the effects of antihypertensive drugs.
6 Tolerance, physical dependence and super-sensitivity.
7 Cholestatic jaundice.
8 Hypothermia; sometimes hyperthermia.
9 Dermatitis.
10 Opacities in lens and cornea.
11 Blood dyscrasias.

Carbimazole: side effects

1 Maculopapular skin rash and urticaria – common side effect.
2 Agranulocytosis. It can present as sore throat and fever and comes a few weeks after the start of the treatment. It is an idiosyncratic effect and thus serial blood counts are of no use. It is transient and can disappear with the withdrawal of the drug.
3 Leukopenia. This too is an idiosyncratic effect and thus serial blood counts are of no use. It is transient and can disappear with the withdrawal of the drug.
4 Goitre. The mechanism is ↓ synthesis of T3 and T4 → ↑ TSH → stimulation of thyroid gland growth.
5 Rare side effects: depigmentation of hair, cholestatic jaundice, lupus-like syndrome, arthralgias and myalgias.

Tetracycline: side effects

1 *Effects on bones and teeth*: Tetracyclines are generally contraindicated during pregnancy. If prescribed, they can cause fetal tooth enamel dysplasia and irregularities in bone growth. Similar ill-effects are produced if tetracyclines are prescribed in children at the time of appearance of permanent teeth.

2 *GIT*:

    a They range from mild NVD to severe, potentially life-threatening enterocolitis.

    b Normal GI flora may be disturbed. This in turn can lead to candidiasis (oral and vaginal) and rarely to bacterial superinfections by *S. aureus* or *Clostridium difficile*.

3 *Hepatotoxicity*: Hepatic necrosis can occur with tetracyclines, especially when given during pregnancy or in patients with pre-existing liver disease.

4 *Nephrotoxicity*: Fanconi's syndrome can occur in patients taking outdated tetracycline. This syndrome is characterised by aminoaciduria, proteinuria and casts in urine. It is because of the formation of a toxic substance – epianhydrotetracycline.

5 *Phototoxicity*: i.e. increased sensitivity to ultraviolet light can occur especially with demeclocycline.

6 *Bone marrow toxicity*: with long-term therapy.

7 *Vestibular toxicity*: in the form of dizziness and vertigo can occur with doxycycline and minocycline. Decreasing the dose can reverse these side effects.

Tetracycline: teratogenicity
TEtracycline is a
TEratogen that causes staining of
TEeth in the newborn.
Teratogenic drugs
'**W/TERATO**genic':
Warfarin
Thalidomide
Epileptic drugs: phenytoin, valproate, carbamazepine
Retinoid
ACE inhibitor
Third element: lithium
OCP and other hormones (e.g. danazol)

Chloramphenicol: side effects

1 *GIT*: NVD, altered taste and superinfections especially candidiasis.

2 *Bone marrow toxicity*:

    a Idiosyncratic aplastic anaemia. It is usually irreversible.

    b Inhibition of red cell maturation $\rightarrow \downarrow$ circulating RBCs. Decreasing the dose can reverse this side effect.

3 *Gray baby syndrome*: Premature neonates who are deficient in glucuronosyl-transferase are particularly prone to develop this syndrome. It is characterised by $\downarrow$ RBS, cyanosis and CV collapse.

4 *Hypersensitivity reactions*: fever, skin rash, optic and peripheral neuritis, enlargement of blind spot and scotoma.

Aminoglycosides: side effects

1 *Ototoxicity – may be irreversible*: Dose of aminoglycosides must be reduced in patients with renal failure. If not, high plasma levels of aminoglycosides can cause auditory or vestibular damage (or both); the damage may be irreversible. Auditory damage primarily occurs with amikacin and kanamycin; vestibular damage primarily occurs

with gentamicin and tobramycin. Concomitant use of loop diuretics increases the chances of development of ototoxicity.

2 *Nephrotoxicity – often reversible*: Acute tubular necrosis (ATN) → proteinuria and appearance of hyaline cats in the urine. Concomitant use of antibiotics (vancomycin; cephalosporins; amphotericin B) increases the chances of development of nephrotoxicity.

3 *NM blockade with respiratory paralysis – rare*: When used in high doses, a curare-like block (due to ↓ presynaptic ACh release and ↓ postsynaptic sensitivity to ACh) can occur with aminoglycosides. It may result in respiratory paralysis. Its antidote is calcium gluconate or neostigmine. Ventilatory support will be required in case of respiratory paralysis.

4 *Contact dermatitis*: can occur in personnel handling the drug especially neomycin.

Phenytoin: therapeutic uses

1 *Anti-epileptic drug*: Phenytoin is effective against all types of epilepsies, e.g. grand mal, psychomotor, focal, cortical, etc. (except absence seizures).

2 *Anti-arrhythmic drug*: Phenytoin is the drug of choice for digitalis-induced arrhythmias as it does not aggravate AV block, rather it facilitates AV conduction.

3 *Miscellaneous*: Various neuralgias, e.g. trigeminal, diabetic neuropathy, chorea, etc.

Phenytoin: side effects

1 Central and peripheral nervous system:
   a Vestibulocerebellar syndrome. This syndrome is characterised by dizziness, nystagmus, ataxia, etc.
   b About 30% of patients show peripheral neuropathy.
   c Ocular toxicity characterised by mydriasis, blurred vision, etc.
   d Behavioural disturbances, e.g. dullness, hallucinations, drowsiness.

2 Gingival hyperplasia characterised by swelling of the gums with or without bleeding.

3 GI upsets (N, V, epigastric distress and anorexia). These can be decreased by taking the drug after meals.

4 Endocrine effects:
   a Decreased or inappropriate release of ADH.
   b Hyperglycemia and glycosuria due to inhibition of insulin secretion.
   c Osteomalacia due to hypocalcemia (as a result of ↓ Ca^{++} absorption from GIT) and biotransformation, turnover and metabolism of vitamins C and K.

5 Hypersensitivity reactions like SLE, Stevens-Johnson's syndrome (SJS) and fatal hepatic necrosis.

6 Hematological reactions like neutropenia, leukopenia, thrombocytopenia, agranulocytosis, ↓ in the RBC count, megaloblastic anaemia, lymphadenopathy (resembling Hodgkin's lymphoma), hyperprothrombinemia in newborns of mothers receiving phenytoin during pregnancy.

7 If high doses of phenytoin are given I/V rapidly, it can cause severe arrhythmias, hypotension and CNS depression.

PHENYTOIN:
P-450 interactions
Hirsutism/**H**ypersensitivity reactions/**H**ematological reactions/**H**yperglycemia and glycosuria

Enlarged gums
Nystagmus
Yellow-browning of skin
Teratogenicity
Osteomalacia
Interference with vitamin B_{12} metabolism ($\rightarrow$ megaloblastic anaemia)
Neuropathies: Vestibulocerebellar syndrome; peripheral neuropathy; ocular toxicity; behavioural disturbances.

Methotrexate: therapeutic uses
1 Used as a disease-modifying antirheumatic drug (DMARD) in rheumatoid arthritis.
2 Anticancer drug: Used in acute lymphocytic leukaemia (ALL), non-Hodgkin's lymphoma, cutaneous T-cell lymphoma, choriocarcinoma and breast cancer.
3 Ectopic pregnancy (methotrexate is an abortifacient).
4 Psoriasis.

Methotrexate: side effects
1 NVD.
2 Mucosal ulcers.
3 Hematotoxicity (bone marrow suppression).
4 Liver toxicity.
5 Renal toxicity.
6 Pulmonary toxicity (in the form of pulmonary infiltrates and fibrosis).
7 Hypersensitivity (it often presents as pneumonitis and is more common in patients with pre-existing pulmonary pathology).
8 In females: menstrual dysfunction.
9 In pregnancy: teratogenicity.
10 Osteoporosis.

Avoidance of side effects
1 Coadministration of folinic acid: The toxic effects of methotrexate on 'normal cells' can be reduced by coadministration of folinic acid (leucovorin). Leucovorin readily accumulates in the normal cells as opposed to the cancerous cells. It bypasses the dihydrofolate reductase step in folic acid synthesis. The net effect is continued synthesis of folic acid despite dihydrofolate reductase inhibition by methotrexate. It is called 'leucovorin rescue'.
2 Advise patient to drink lot of water. This is because methotrexate gets excreted unchanged via kidneys. If adequate hydration status is not maintained, methotrexate can precipitate in the renal tubules.

Cyclophosphamide: therapeutic uses
1 It is used in autoimmune disease like autoimmune hemolytic anaemia, autoimmune red-cell aplasia.
2 In bone marrow transplant patients. However, it does not prevent GVH (graft vs host) reaction.
3 Anticancer uses include non-Hodgkin's lymphoma, acute lymphocytic leukaemia (ALL), breast CA, ovarian CA and neuroblastoma.

Cyclophosphamide: side effects

1 Bone marrow suppression ($\rightarrow$ pancytopenia).
2 Haemorrhagic cystitis. It is caused by one of the break down products of cyclophosphamide called acrolein. This side effect can be avoided by concomitant use of mercaptoethanesulfonate (mesna) and advising the patient to take lot of drinking water. Mesna 'traps' acrolein and thus reduces the incidence of haemorrhagic cystitis – an example of 'rescue therapy'.
3 Sterility.
4 Alopecia.
5 Cardiac dysfunction.
6 Pulmonary toxicity.
7 Syndrome of inappropriate antidiuretic hormone secretion (SIADH).
8 NVD.

Doxorubicin and daunorubicin: side effects

1 Bone marrow suppression ($\rightarrow$ pancytopenia).
2 The most distinctive side effect of these anthracyclines is cardiotoxicity (arrhythmias; cardiomyopathy; CHF). It can be avoided by 'rescue therapy' with dexrazoxane. As we know that anthracyclines generate free radicals, which in turn block the synthesis of RNA and DNA. Dexrazoxane administration inhibits free radical formation and thus prevents cardiotoxicity.
3 Alopecia.
4 NVD.

Amphotericin B: therapeutic uses

1 *As an I/V infusion*: Amongst all the antifungals, amphotericin B has the widest spectrum of activity. It is used for a variety of systemic fungal infections caused by Aspergillus, Blastomyces, Candida albicans, Cryptococcus, Histoplasma and Mucor.
2 *Intrathecal infusion* for fungal meningitis. Intrathecal infusion is dangerous as it can lead to neurotoxicity in the form of neurological damage and seizures.
3 *Topically*: For mycotic corneal ulcers and keratitis.

Nystatin: therapeutic uses

1 Oral candidiasis.
2 Oesophageal candidiasis (in immunocompromised patients).

Griseofulvin: therapeutic uses

1 Dermatophytosis of skin and hair.

Metoclopramide: therapeutic uses

1 To prevent NV due to gastroduodenal, hepatic and biliary diseases.
2 Used in some patients with non-ulcer dyspepsia.
3 Gastro-esophageal reflux.
4 In post-op conditions.
5 In high doses to prevent NV associated with cytotoxic drug therapy/radiotherapy.
6 Used in radiology for speeding the transit of barium during intestinal follow-through examination.

Metoclopramide: side effects
1 Extrapyramidal side effects (tremors; rigidity; bradykinesia). The classical symptoms of Parkinsonism are the same (i.e. tremors; rigidity; bradykinesia).
2 Drowsiness.
3 Hyperprolactinemia.

Sodium nitroprusside: therapeutic uses
1 It is only used in hypertensive emergencies as an intravenous infusion.

Sodium nitroprusside: side effects
1 Excessive hypotension.
2 Tachycardia.
3 When infusion is continued for several days, it can lead to accumulation of cyanide/thiocyanate in the blood.

Oxytocin: therapeutic uses
1 Induction/augmentation of labour.
2 Post-partum uterine haemorrhage.
3 Incomplete abortion.
4 Impaired milk ejection.
5 Oxytocin challenge test (to know placental circulatory reservoirs). An abnormal response suggests intrauterine growth retardation and may require immediate caesarean delivery.

Prostaglandins (PGs): therapeutic uses
1 Facilitation of labour at term (softening of cervix).
2 Induction of labour.
3 Abortifacient (vaginal suppository or oral dinoprostone, mifepristone).

Ergometrine: therapeutic uses
1 PPH (if oxytocin is ineffective to control atonic uterus). Dose: 150–250 microgram I/V.

Aluminium hydroxide: therapeutic uses
1 Peptic ulcer disease.
2 Hyperphosphatemia in renal impairment.

Sucralfate: therapeutic uses
1 Peptic ulcer disease.
2 Upper GI bleeding in critically ill patients.
3 Prevention of stress-related bleeding.

Misoprostol: therapeutic uses
1 NSAID-induced peptic ulcers (incidence 20% is reduced to 3%).

Colloidal bismuth compounds: therapeutic uses
1 Peptic ulcer disease.
2 Eradication of *H. Pylori*.
3 Traveller's diarrhoea.

5

Drug differences

Table 5.1 **Differences between atropine and hyoscine**

	Atropine	*Hyoscine*
Source:	Atropa belladonna and Dhatura stramonium	Hyoscyamus niger and Scopolia canolica
Chemistry:	Ester of tropic acid and tropine	Ester of tropic acid and scopine
Mechanism of action:	Antimuscarinic, competitive antagonist of acetylcholine	Antimuscarinic, competitive antagonist of acetylcholine
Duration of action:	Prolong	Short
Peripheral antimuscarinic action:	More prominent on heart, GIT and bronchial muscle	More prominent on eyes, salivary and bronchial secretion and sweat
Action on CNS:	Stimulation, followed by depression	Depression from the beginning (in the presence of pain, there may be excitement)
Loss of memory:	Not seen	It causes amnesia to recent events. It is thus more commonly used as a pre-anaesthetic medication as compared to atropine
Motion sickness and Parkinsonism:	Less useful	More useful
Toxicity:	Restlessness, excitement, mania and delirium	Drowsiness
Dose:	0.25–2 mg	0.3–0.6 mg

Table 5.2 Differences between non-opioids (NSAIDs) and opioids

	Non-opioids (NSAIDs)	Opioids
Source:	Synthetic	Natural opium alkaloids/semi-synthetic/synthetic morphine substitutes
Structure:	Heterogeneous	Phenanthrene compounds, benzyl-isoquinoline compounds
Type of pain relieved:	Somatic pain arising from musculoskeletal structures	Deep visceral pain
Mechanism of action:	• Inhibition of prostaglandin synthesis by inhibiting the cyclo-oxygenase enzyme • Inhibits generation of nociception by inhibiting the peripheral nociceptors • No action on specific opioid receptors (μ, κ, δ, ε, σ)	• Decreased nociception input, decreased processing and integration, decreased transmission, decreased perception and decreased emotional reaction to pain. Decreased release of neurotransmitters (especially excitatory neurotransmitters like glutamic acid). By causing hyper-polarisation due to increase in potassium efflux • Acts on opioid receptors (μ, κ, δ, ε, σ)
CNS devpression:	Do not depress CNS	Depress CNS

(continued)

Table 5.2 Differences between non-opioids (NSAIDs) and opioids (continued)

	Non-opioids (NSAIDs)	Opioids
Pharmacological actions and effects:	• Acts as analgesics, antipyretic, anti-inflammatory, antiplatelet (at low doses) and uricosuric (at high doses) • No antispasmodic effect on GIT smooth muscles (unlike morphine which commonly causes constipation, NSAIDs do not cause constipation)	• Acts only as analgesics. Also produce euphoria, sedation, hypnosis and cough suppression. No antipyretic and anti-inflammatory effects • Morphine-like alkaloids produce constipation through decreased intestinal peristalsis which is mediated by effects on opioids receptors in the enteric nervous system. Hence clinically used as antidiarrhoeal agents • Also opioids alone produce contraction of sphincter pupillae (→ miosis), truncal rigidly, contraction of biliary smooth muscle (→ biliary colic), contraction of sphincter of Oddi (reflux of biliary and pancreatic secretion) and relaxation of uterine smooth muscle (→ prolongation of labour)
Tolerance and dependence:	Do not produce tolerance/dependence	Produce tolerance/dependence
Withdrawal syndrome:	Do not produce withdrawal syndrome	Produce withdrawal syndrome
Side effects:	Mainly due to inhibition of prostaglandin synthesis like peptic ulceration, upper GI bleed, bleeding tendency, precipitation of an acute attack of asthma (due to ↑ synthesis of leukotrienes), Reye's syndrome (hepatic fatty degeneration and encephalopathy), ARF, interstitial nephritis, respiratory alkalosis (at high doses) and metabolic acidosis (at toxic doses)	Mainly due to CNS depression. Most serious is depression of the respiratory centre; others include ↑ ICP, postural hypotension, urinary retention, constipation, itching around nose and urticaria

Table 5.3 **Differences between morphine and pethidine**

	Morphine	*Pethidine*
Source:	Natural	Synthetic
Chemistry:	Phenanthrene derivative	Phenylpiperidine derivative
Pharmacokinetics:	• Route of administration: S/C, I/M, I/V, epidural, intrathecal and per-rectal • Bioavailability: 25% • Plasma protein binding: 33% • Onset of action: slow • Duration of action: longer (3–5hrs)	• Route of administration: Oral, S/C, I/M • Bioavailability: 50% • Plasma protein binding: 60% • Onset of action: quick • Duration of action: short (2–4hrs)
Metabolism:	Glucuronidation in liver	Demethylation in liver
Metabolites:	Morphine-3-glucuronide and Morphine-6-glucuronide. Both metabolites are active	Normepridine ($\rightarrow$ CNS stimulation; but no analgesic property)
Pharmaco-dynamics:	• Receptors: µ predominantly • Potency: more as analgesic • Sedation: more marked • Miosis: present • Corneal anaesthesia and loss of corneal reflex: absent • Bronchoconstriction: present • Cough suppression: present • Effect on heart rate: bradycardia • Antimuscarinic effects: absent • Spasmogenic effect: present • Urinary retention: present • Constipation: more marked • Pregnancy and lactation: contraindicated because morphine delays labour • Withdrawal syndrome: long-lived (8–10 days)	• Receptors: κ predominantly • Potency: 1/10th as analgesic • Sedation: less marked • Miosis: absent • Corneal anaesthesia and loss of corneal reflex: present (on parenteral administration) • Bronchoconstriction: absent • Cough suppression: absent • Effect on heart rate: tachycardia • Antimuscarinic effects: present • Spasmogenic effect: absent • Urinary retention: absent • Constipation: less marked • Pregnancy and lactation: can be given (no effect on labour) • Withdrawal syndrome: short-lived (4–6 days)
Therapeutic uses:	Analgesic, LVF with massive pulmonary oedema, pre-anaesthetic medication and anxiety	Analgesic (for short procedures like upper/lower GI endoscopy, cystoscopy, I/V ascending pyelography)
Excretion:	Not affected by acidification of urine	Acidification of urine increases excretion

Table 5.4 **Differences between heparin and warfarin**

	Heparin	*Warfarin*
Source:	Bovine lungs, porcine intestinal mucosa	Semi-synthetic
Chemistry:	Mucopolysaccharide	Coumarin derivative
Structure:	Large polymer, acidic	Small, lipid-soluble
Route of administration:	Parenteral (S/C, I/V)	Oral
Site of action:	Blood	Liver
Mechanism of action:	It binds to antithrombin-III (ATIII) forming a heparin-ATIII complex. This complex binds and irreversibly inactivates thrombin (activated factor II), factors IXa, Xa, XIa, XIIa, and XIIIa. In the presence of heparin, ATIII proteolyses clotting factors 1000-fold faster than in its absence	Warfarin inhibits Vit-K dependent synthesis of factors X, VII, IX and X in the liver by inhibiting the enzyme Vit-K epoxide reductase
Onset of action:	Quick (in seconds). Since heparin acts by inactivating the pre-formed clotting factors, it produces its therapeutic effect immediately	Slow (36–48hrs). Since warfarin acts by inhibiting the synthesis of clotting factors, its therapeutic effect is produced only when the pre-formed clotting factors having t½ of 8–60hrs are eliminated from the circulation. Also, whereas effect of warfarin can be reversed by giving Vit-K, it only occurs when Vit-K causes the synthesis of new clotting factors – a process that takes 6–24hrs. More rapid reversal requires transfusion of fresh frozen plasma (FFP) that contains normal clotting factors
Effect on vascular tone:	Vasodilatation	Nil
Duration of action:	Short (10–15 min)	Long (4–7 days)
Protein binding:	Nil	Extensive
Metabolites:	Uroheparin	S-warfarin-7-hydroxy warfarin; R-warfarin-warfarin alcohol
Half-life:	40–90 min	15–70hrs

(*continued*)

	Heparin	Warfarin
Therapeutic uses:	Used when anticoagulation is needed immediately, i.e. on starting anticoagulant therapy, heparin is given first, followed 24hrs later by warfarin. Important therapeutic indications include DVT, pulmonary embolism, acute MI (in combination with thrombolytics for revascularisation), atrial fibrillation, coronary angioplasty and placement of coronary stents (in combination with glycoprotein IIb/IIIa inhibitors), CVA, haemodialysis/peritoneal dialysis, anticoagulation during pregnancy and to preserve blood in vitro	Warfarin is used for chronic anticoagulation (starting 24hrs after commencement of heparin therapy) in all of the clinical situations described for heparin (except during pregnancy). Heparin-warfarin combination therapy is continued for 4–5 days, followed by warfarin monotherapy for months or may be more depending upon the indication
Pregnancy and lactation:	Safe	Contraindicated (teratogenic: causes bone defects and multiple haemorrhages in the developing fetus)
Adverse effects:	Bleeding (commonest side effect), thrombocytopenia, osteoporosis, transient alopecia, allergic reactions (like asthma, urticaria and anaphylactic shock)	Bleeding (commonest side effect), teratogenicity, decreased production of Protein C ($\rightarrow$ development of a period of hypercoagulability; heparin is thus always started before warfarin therapy to avoid the development of hypercoagulability)
Drug interactions:	Nil	Cytochrome P450-inducing drugs $\rightarrow \uparrow$ warfarin clearance $\rightarrow \downarrow$ anticoagulant effect. Cytochrome P450-inhibiting drugs $\rightarrow \downarrow$ warfarin clearance $\rightarrow \uparrow$ anticoagulant effect
Antidote:	Protamine sulphate 1% I/V is the antidote for unfractionated heparin; it only partially reverses the effects of LMW heparins	Vit K (phytomenadione) I/V

Table 5.5 **Differences between cimetidine and ranitidine**

	Cimetidine	*Ranitidine*
Chemistry:	Imidazole derivative	Furan derivative
Duration of action:	Short (4–6hrs)	Long (8–12hrs)
Bioavailability:	60%	50%
Plasma protein binding:	20%	15%
Binding with cytochrome P450:	Present	Negligible
Increase in cell-mediated immunity:	Yes	No
Hepatic blood flow:	Decreased	Decreased
Crossing of blood brain barrier (BBB):	Poor	Very poor
Potency:	Less	5–10 times more potent
Elimination t½:	2–3hrs	2–3hrs
Drug interactions:	Interferes with hepatic metabolism of drugs like digoxin, warfarin, benzodiazepines, beta-blockers, etc.	Negligible
Toxicity:	CNS: lethargy, hallucinations, convulsions Endocrine: Unlike ranitidine, cimetidine causes hyperprolactinemia ($\rightarrow$ gynecomastia in males and galactorrhea in females) Hepatotoxicity: As compared to ranitidine, cimetidine is a potent inhibitor of hepatic drug metabolising enzyme (CYP450)	Endocrine: Doesn't cause hyperprolactinemia. Hepatotoxicity: Less potent inhibitor of hepatic drug metabolising enzyme (CYP450)
Dose:	800 mg/day in divided doses	300 mg/day in divided doses

Table 5.6 **Differences between adrenaline and noradrenaline**

	Adrenaline	*Noradrenaline*
Source:	Adrenal medulla	Postganglionic sympathetic nerve endings
Chemistry:	Catecholamine (contains methyl group)	Catecholamine (does not contain methyl group)
Receptors stimulated:	$\alpha1$, $\alpha2$, $\beta1$, $\beta2$, $\beta3$	$\alpha1$, $\alpha2$, $\beta1$
Effects on the cardiovascular system:	Rate: ↑ • Force of contraction: ↑ • Excitability and conductivity: much increased • Coronary blood flow: ↑ • Cardiac output: ↑ • Arteriolar tone in the skeletal muscles: vasodilatation • Arteriolar tone in skin and viscera: vasoconstriction • Total peripheral resistance: ↓ • Systolic blood pressure: ↑ • Diastolic blood pressure: ↓	Rate: ↓ • Force of contraction: little effect • Excitability and conductivity: increased • Coronary blood flow: ↑ • Cardiac output: no change or ↓ • Arteriolar tone in the skeletal muscles: vasoconstriction • Arteriolar tone in skin and viscera: vasoconstriction • Total peripheral resistance: ↑ • Systolic blood pressure: ↑ • Diastolic blood pressure: ↑
Effects on smooth muscles:	• Intestine and bladder: relax • Bronchi: relax • Sphincter: constrict • Uterus: inhibition of uterine contraction • Eye: mydriasis	• Intestine and bladder: relax • Bronchi: little effect • Sphincter: constrict • Uterus: stimulation of uterine contraction • Eye: mydriasis
Metabolism (glycogenolysis and O_2 consumption):	↑	Insignificant effect

Table 5.7 **Differences between methyl dopa and clonidine**

	Methyldopa	*Clonidine*
Structure:	Structural analogue to levodopa	2-imidazole derivative
Mechanism of action:	It is a pro-drug. After having been converted to alpha-methyl-norepinephrine, it acts as an agonist on the postsynaptic $\alpha2$-receptors in the CNS $\rightarrow \downarrow$ sympathetic outflow from the centre to periphery	It is an active drug that acts as an agonist on the postsynaptic $\alpha2$-receptors in the CNS $\rightarrow \downarrow$ sympathetic outflow from the centre to periphery
Pharmacokinetics:	On oral administration, absorption is incomplete and slow with extensive first-pass metabolism. Elimination is mainly through liver metabolism and some through renal excretion	Being lipid-soluble, GI absorption of clonidine is rapid. Elimination is mainly through renal excretion
Route of administration:	Oral, sometimes I/V in emergencies	Oral and transdermal (I the form of patch), but never I/V
T½	2hrs	8–12hrs
Bioavailability:	25%	95%
Dose-response curved:	Increasing doses are not more effective	Increasing doses are more effective (and also more toxic)
Reduction in dosage required in moderate renal insufficiency:	No	Yes
Pharmacologic effects:	It reduces blood pressure chiefly by reducing peripheral vascular resistance	It reduces blood pressure both by reducing heart rate (and thus cardiac output) and peripheral vascular resistance
Therapeutic uses:	Mild to moderate cases of hypertension, hypertensive crisis and carcinoid syndrome	Mild to moderate cases of hypertension, diabetic diarrhoea ($\rightarrow \uparrow$ Na^+ and H_2O reabsorption and $\downarrow$ secretion of HCO_3) and alcohol/tobacco/opioid withdrawal syndrome. It is contraindicated in hypertensive crisis

(*continued*)

139

	Methyldopa	Clonidine
Toxicity:	Causes sedation (commonest side effect), extrapyramidal signs (Parkinsonism), ↑ prolactin secretion (→ lactation), positive Coomb's test, hemolytic anaemia, hepatitis and drug fever	Common side effects include sedation and dry mouth. It also causes depression. In case depression develops during the course of the therapy, clonidine should be withdrawn. If withdrawn suddenly after protracted use, clonidine can precipitate hypertensive crisis. It should, therefore, be withdrawn gradually. In case hypertensive crisis develops, it is treated by reinstitution of clonidine or administration of α- and β-blockers

6

Miscellaneous

Halothane
Advantages
1 Good physical properties.
2 Used to produce controlled hypotension and bloodless field during plastic/vascular surgery.
3 Potent anaesthetic.
4 Produces bronchodilatation (useful in asthmatic patients).
5 Potent relaxant of masseter muscles.
6 Potent inhibitor of laryngeal and pharyngeal reflexes.
7 Does not cause bronchospasm, laryngospasm and coughing.

Disadvantages
1 Poor analgesic.
2 Poor muscle relaxant.
3 Profound hypotension, if given in more than 2% concentration.
4 Increases para-sympathetic tone, leading to bradycardia.
5 Sensitises ventricular muscle and conduction tissue to adrenaline, causing arrhythmias.
6 Hepatotoxic and respiratory depressant.
7 Expensive, and special apparatus is needed for administration.
8 Can cause malignant hyperthermia (ryanodine receptors).
9 Genetic mutations $\rightarrow$ more binding of Ca^{++} with the receptors.

Nitrous oxide
Advantages
1 Rapid induction and recovery.
2 Non-inflammable, non-irritating and non-explosive (however supports combustion).
3 Very potent analgesic (30–40% analgesia; 65–70% loss of consciousness; and 80% plane 1 of surgical anaesthesia).
4 Used in procedures of short duration (tooth-extraction, obstetrical analgesia, cleansing and debridement of wounds and cauterisation).
5 Induction and maintenance of anaesthesia, along with I/V thiopentone-gas-oxygen-halothane technique called balanced-anaesthesia.
6 Safe. No organ toxicity (respiratory, renal, CVS, or hepatic).
7 Measurement of cerebral and coronary blood flow by Fick's Principle.

8 Decreases the dose of general anaesthetic. When combined → decreased complications and decreased recovery period from anaesthesia.

Disadvantages

1 Not a potent anaesthetic and muscle relaxant, so violent excitement can occur.
2 Second gas effect leading to transient hypoxia.
3 CO_2 accumulation and hypoxia→ cardiac irregularities during anaesthesia.
4 Specialised apparatus to control its administration.
5 Administration for more than 7 hours, leads to bone-marrow depression (leukopenia and anaemia).
6 Prolonged administration → peripheral neuropathy, megaloblastic anaemia (due to interference with vitamin B_{12} metabolism) and abortion.

Ketamine
Advantages

1 Effective by both intravenous and intramuscular routes.
2 Anaesthesia is accompanied by profound analgesia.
3 Does not produce vomiting, hypotension and bronchospasm.
4 Less respiratory complications, due to less impairment of laryngeal/pharyngeal reflexes.
5 Useful for poor risk geriatric/elderly and unstable patients.
6 Used in low doses, as outpatient anaesthesia.

Disadvantages

1 No muscle relaxation.
2 Tends to raise heart rate, intraocular and intracranial pressures.
3 Cannot be used for surgery on larynx, pharynx and bronchi.
4 Poor in relieving visceral pain.
5 Emergence phenomenon (characterised by bad dreams, post-op disorientation and sensory/perceptual delusions). Its Rx is diazepam, before the operation.

Thiopentone sodium
Advantages

1 Ease of administration.
2 Non-explosive.
3 Induction and recovery is rapid and pleasant.
4 No irritation of mucous membranes.
5 No sensitisation of myocardium to adrenaline.
6 No/less incidence of post-op vomiting and excitement.
7 Low incidence of post-anaesthetic complications.

Disadvantages

1 Stages of anaesthesia cannot be recognised.
2 Pupils remain normal or constricted.
3 During induction, unpleasant and fatal reactions (like apnea, coughing, hiccough, laryngospasm and bronchospasm) may develop.
4 Depression of myocardium, respiratory and vasomotor centres.
5 Rapid injection can lead to hypotension and cardiac arrhythmias.

6 Intra-arterial injection→ severe pain and gangrene.

7 Inadequate muscle relaxation.

8 Laryngeal and pharyngeal reflexes are not abolished.

9 Regurgitation due to relaxation of gastro-esophageal sphincter.

10 Injury to surrounding nerves and tissues.

11 Thromboembolism.

12 Can precipitate porphyria in susceptible individuals.

Preference of benzodiazepines over barbiturates

1 High margin of safety (i.e. 10 times the normal dose can be given without harmful effects).

2 Least drug interactions, since no effect on the drug metabolising cytochrome P450 enzyme system in the liver.

3 Selectivity of action (i.e. like barbiturates, benzodiazepines are not a general CNS depressant – they act mainly on limbic system).

4 Lack of interactions (i.e. neither enzyme inhibitors nor enzyme inducers).

5 Do not cause hyperalgesia.

6 Fewer incidences of drug dependence/addiction.

7 Less severe withdrawal syndrome.

8 Less severe tolerance.

9 Least alteration in sleep pattern.

Digoxin toxicity: features

1 Arrhythmias (especially AV block).

2 Nausea, vomiting, diarrhoea.

3 Headache; dizziness.

4 Seizures.

5 Xanthopsia (yellow vision).

6 Skin reactions.

7 Impotence.

Digoxin toxicity: causes

1 Electrolyte disturbances ($\downarrow$ K$^+$; $\downarrow$ Mg^{++}; $\uparrow$ Ca^{++}).

2 Renal impairment.

3 Hypothyroidism.

4 Drug-induced (ACEI[7]; Ca-channel blockers; amiodarone[8]; quinidine; cyclosporine).

Digoxin toxicity: management

- Prevent absorption: gastric lavage; activated charcoal (if patient comes within 6–8hrs of ingestion).
- Correct electrolyte disturbances ($\downarrow$ K$^+$; $\downarrow$ Mg^{++}; $\uparrow$ Ca^{++}). K$^+$ should not be raised above the level of 5 mEq/L.
  - For bradyarrhythmia: Atropine.
  - For symptomatic bradycardia that has failed to respond to atropine: Temporary pacemaker.

---

7 ACEI reduce renal clearance of digoxin → digoxin toxicity.

8 Amiodarone displaces digoxin from the binding proteins → digoxin toxicity.

- For supraventricular tachycardia (SVT): Verapamil.
- For ventricular tachycardia (VT): Lignocaine; phenytoin.

Digoxin toxicity: indications of digoxin-binding antibody fragment[9]

1 Reserved for very severe cases:
- Patients who have taken a large overdose (≥10 mg in adults and ≥4 mg in children).
- Serum digoxin level >13 nmol/L.
- Serum K+ level >5 mmol/L.
- Presence of life-threatening arrhythmias (2nd or 3rd degree AV block; VT; VF).

Aspirin/salicylate toxicity

It could be mild (called salicylism) or severe.

Mild toxicity: features
- GI: N, V.
- Respiratory: Hyperventilation (salicylate toxicity → metabolic acidosis → hyperventilation).
- CNS: Headache; dizziness; tinnitus (ringing of ears).

Severe toxicity: features

Symptoms of mild toxicity are followed by restlessness, delirium, hallucinations, convulsions and coma. The usual cause of death is respiratory failure.

Lethal dose

In children: ≥10 gm
In adults: 300 mg/kg

Investigations

1 Serum salicylate levels (levels of >70 mg/dl indicate severe intoxication).
2 Arterial blood gases (to determine pH): It will initially show respiratory alkalosis (d/t hyperventilation) followed by metabolic acidosis (d/t drug itself).

Treatment

Mild cases:
1 Symptomatic.
2 Alkaline diuresis (NaHCO3 added in dextrose water → alkalisation of urine → increasing the urinary pH enhances the elimination of salicylate).

Severe cases:
1 Haemodialysis.
2 Mechanical ventilation (if pulmonary oedema develops).
3 Intravenous mannitol (if cerebral oedema develops).

Acetaminophen (paracetamol) toxicity

Acetaminophen is acted upon by cytochrome P450 mixed-function oxidase to form a toxic intermediate (called *N*-acetyl-*p*-benzoquinoneimine). In therapeutic doses, this

---

9 Normally given as I/V infusion over 30 minutes. In cases of cardiac arrest, it can be given as I/V bolus. It freely filters through the kidneys and thus can be given even in CRF patients.

toxic intermediate conjugates with hepatic glutathione to form non-toxic mercapturic acid. In lethal doses, all available glutathione reserves of the liver are depleted and the toxic intermediate combines with the essential hepatic cell proteins, resulting in cell death/hepatic necrosis – a potentially life-threatening condition (renal tubular necrosis can also occur → acute renal failure).

In patients who are already suffering from some chronic liver disease, the glutathione reserves may be subnormal so that even near-normal doses of paracetamol may cause hepatic necrosis.

Treatment
If given within 10 hours of paracetamol toxicity, N-acetylcysteine, which contains sulfhydryl groups to which the toxic intermediate can bind, is life-saving.

7

Important tables

Table 7.1 Important receptors and their agonists and antagonists

Receptor	Agonist/s	Antagonist/s
5-HT$_2$-receptor	5-Hydroxytryptamine	Ketanserine
D$_2$-receptor	Dopamine Bromocriptine	Chlorpromazine
Mu (μ) receptor	Morphine	Naloxone
β-adrenoceptor	Noradrenaline Isoprenaline	Propranolol
Nicotinic ACh receptor	Acetylcholine Nicotine	Tubocurarine
H$_1$-receptor	Histamine	Mepyramine
H$_2$-receptor	Impromidine	Cimetidine Ranitidine
Insulin receptor	Insulin	Not known
Oestrogen receptor	Ethinylestradiol	Tamoxifen
Progesterone receptor	Norethisterone	Danazol

Table 7.2 Main effects of autonomic nervous system

Structure	Parasympathetic effect	Receptor involved	Sympathetic effect	Receptor involved
Eye: pupils	Constriction	M_3	Dilatation	α
Eye: ciliary muscle	Contraction	M_3	Relaxation	β
Lacrimal gland	Secretion	M_3	No effect	–
Salivary glands	Secretion (we salivate when we are about to eat)	M_3	No effect	α, β
Skin: sweat glands	No effect	–	Secretion (when we fight, we sweat)	α
Skin: pilomotor	No effect	–	Piloerection	α
Airways	Constriction	M_3	Dilatation	β_2
Mast cells			Inhibition of histamine release	β_2
SA node	↓ Heart rate	M_2	↑ Heart rate	β_1
AV node	Speed of conduction slowed	M_2	Speed of conduction made fast	β_1
Myocardium	↓ Force of contraction (only atria affected; ventricles spared)	M_2	↑ Force of contraction (both atria and ventricles affected)	β_1

(continued)

Table 7.2 Main effects of autonomic nervous system (continued)

Structure	Parasympathetic effect	Receptor involved	Sympathetic effect	Receptor involved
Arterioles: • Brain • Coronary • Cutaneous • Erectile tissue • Salivary glands • Skeletal muscles • Visceras	Except arterioles of erectile tissue and salivary glands, which are dilated, parasympathetic system does not affect arterioles elsewhere	M_3	Sympathetic system affects all arteriolar beds mentioned on the left. It causes dilatation of the skeletal muscle arterioles. At rest of the places it causes constriction	It is α-receptor everywhere, except skeletal muscles where β_2 receptors are stimulated
Veins	No effect	–	Constriction Dilatation	α β_2
Platelets			Aggregation	α_2
GI smooth muscles	↑ Motility	M_3	↓ Motility	$\alpha_1, \alpha_2, \beta_2$
GI sphincters	Dilatation	M_3	Constriction	α_2, β_2
GI glands	Secretion	M_3	No effect	–
Gastric acid secretion	↑	M_1	No effect	
Pancreatic islets secretion	↑ Insulin secretion		↓ Insulin secretion	α_2
Liver	No effect	–	↑ Glucose output (by ↑ glycogenolysis and gluconeogenesis)	α_1, β_2
Kidney	No effect	–	Renin secretion (when we fight, body tries to conserve the water)	β_2

(continued)

Structure	Parasympathetic effect	Receptor involved	Sympathetic effect	Receptor involved
Pregnant uterus	Variable	–	Contraction (when pregnant ladies get tense, they start having birth pains)	α_1
Non-pregnant uterus	No effect	–	Relaxation	β_2
Penis	Erection	M_3	Ejaculation	α
Bladder detrusor	Contraction		Relaxation	β_2
Bladder sphincter	Relaxation		Contraction	α_1

Table 7.3 **Important ion channels and their stimulators and blockers**

Ion channel	Stimulator/s	Blocker/s
GABA-gated Cl⁻ channel	Benzodiazepines	Picrotoxin
Renal tubular Na⁺ channel	Aldosterone	K⁺-sparing diuretics (amiloride, etc.)
Voltage-gated Na⁺ channel	Veratridine	Local anaesthetics
Voltage-gated Ca⁺⁺ channel	Dihydropyridines β-agonists	–
ATP-sensitive K⁺ channel	Sulphonylureas	ATP

Table 7.4 **Important enzyme-inhibiting drugs**

Drug	Enzyme inhibited
Acetazolamide	Carbonic anhydrase
Aciclovir	Thymidine kinase
Allopurinol	Xanthine oxidase
Anti-HIV drugs (didanosine and zidovudine)	Reverse transcriptase
Aspirin	Cyclooxygenase (COX)
Captopril	ACE
Carbidopa	Dopa decarboxylase
Heparin	Enzymes involved in blood clotting cascade
Methotrexate	Dihydrofolate reductase
Neostigmine	Acetylcholinesterase
Organophosphorous compounds	Acetylcholinesterase
Selegiline	MAO-B
Simvastatin	HMG-CoA reductase
Trimethoprim	Dihydrofolate reductase

Table 7.5 Important drugs that inhibit transport proteins

Drug	Transport protein inhibited
Cocaine	5HT and α_2 presynaptic receptors ($\rightarrow$ inhibition of reuptake of serotonin and noradrenaline respectively)
Tricyclic antidepressants	5HT and α_2 presynaptic receptors ($\rightarrow$ inhibition of reuptake of serotonin and noradrenaline respectively)
Digoxin	Na^+/K^+ ATPase pump ($\rightarrow$ $\uparrow$ force of contraction, $\downarrow$ rate of AV nodal conduction)
Loop diuretics	$Na^+/K^+/Cl^-$ co-transporter (along the thick ascending limb [TAL] of loop of Henle) $\rightarrow$ inhibition of NaCl reabsorption
Omeprazole	H^+/K^+-ATPase proton pump (along the luminal surface of gastric parietal cells) $\rightarrow$ total inhibition of HCl synthesis
Probenecid	Weak acid carrier (along the proximal convoluted tubule [PCT]) $\rightarrow$ inhibition of urate absorption from the PCT

Table 7.6 Important drugs that undergo extensive first-pass metabolism

CVS drugs:
- Aspirin
- Nitrates (GTN; isosorbide dinitrate)
- Metoprolol
- Propranolol
- Verapamil

Respiratory drugs:
- Salbutamol

CNS drugs:
- Levodopa
- Morphine

Table 7.7 Important drugs that produce active metabolites

Drug	Active/toxic metabolite
Azathioprine	Mercaptopurine
Cortisone	Hydrocortisone
Diazepam	Oxazepam
Enalapril	Enalaprilat
Morphine	Morphine 6-glucuronide
Prednisone	Prednisolone

Table 7.8 Important drugs that produce toxic metabolites

Drug	Active/toxic metabolite
Cyclophosphamide	Acrolein
Halothane	Trifluoroacetic acid
Paracetamol	N-acetyl-p-benzoquinone imine

Table 7.9 Drugs that are excreted primarily unchanged in urine

CVS:
- Atenolol
- Frusemide
- Digoxin

ANS:
- Neostigmine

Antibiotics:
- Benzylpenicillin
- Gentamicin
- Oxytetracycline

Immunomodulator:
- Methotrexate

Index

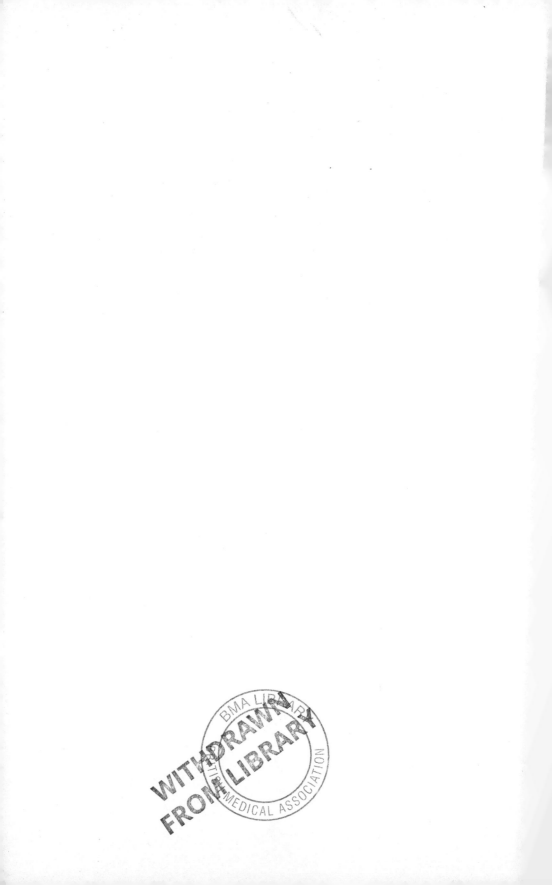